How to Lose 4
30 Days w

SPECIAL EDITION

How To Lose Weight Fast, Keep it Off & Renew
The Mind, Body & Spirit Through Fasting, Smart
Eating & Practical Spirituality - Volume 7

ROBERT DAVE JOHNSTON

How to Lose 40 Pounds (Or More) in 30 Days With Water Fasting

Published by:

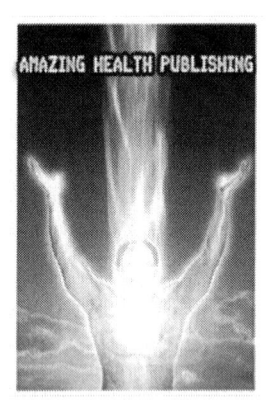

Copyright

Copyright © 2012, Robert Dave Johnston, Amazing Health Publishing. Cover and internal design © Robert Dave Johnston. All rights reserved. No part of this book may be reproduced in any form or by any electronic or mechanical means including information storage and retrieval systems – except in the case of brief quotations in articles or reviews – without the permission in writing from its publisher, Amazing Horror Publishing/Robert Dave Johnston. All of the people, places and things depicted in this book are fictional. Any resemblance to a real person, place or otherwise is totally coincidental.

Disclaimer & Legal Notices

The health-related information and suggestions contained in any of the books or written material mentioned above are based on the research, experience and opinions of the Author and other contributors. Nothing herein should be misinterpreted as actual medical advice, such as one would obtain from a Physician, or as advice for self-diagnosis or as any manner of prescription for self-treatment.

Neither is any information herein to be considered a particular or general cure for any ailment, disease or other health issue. The material contained within is offered strictly and solely for the purpose of providing Holistic health education to the general public. Persons with any health condition should consult a medical professional before entering this or any fasting, weight loss, detoxification or health related program.

Even if you suffer from no known illness, we recommend that you seek medical advice before starting any fasting, weight loss and/or detoxification program, and before choosing to follow any advice given this book. For any products or services mentioned or suggested in this book, you should read all packaging and instructions, as no substance, natural or drug, can be guaranteed to work in everyone. Information and statements regarding dietary supplements, products or services mentioned in this book many not have been evaluated by the Food and Drug Administration and are not intended to diagnose, treat, cure, or prevent any disease. Never disregard or delay in seeking professional medical advice because of something you have read in this book.

Nothing that you read in this book should be regarded as medical or health advice. If you do anything recommended in this book, without the supervision of a licensed medical doctor, you do so at your own risk. Not recommended for persons with any health related condition unless supervised by a qualified health practitioner.

Because there is always some risk involved in any health-related program, the Author, Publisher and contributors assume no responsibility for any adverse effects or consequences resulting from the use of any suggested preparations or procedures described in any of the books or other written materials associated with the website FitnessThroughFasting.com. The author reserves the right to alter and update his opinions based on new conditions at any time.

Dedication

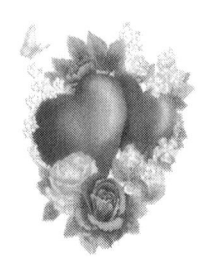

This series of books are dedicated to my mother Sonia Noemi, without whom I would not even be alive today. I love you mom. Thank you for never losing faith in me and supporting me, even when everything seemed hopeless and everyone else had given up on me. I owe you everything. I could collect all of the precious stones on this earth and lay them on your lap, and even still, I would not even come close to giving back to you all that you have given me.

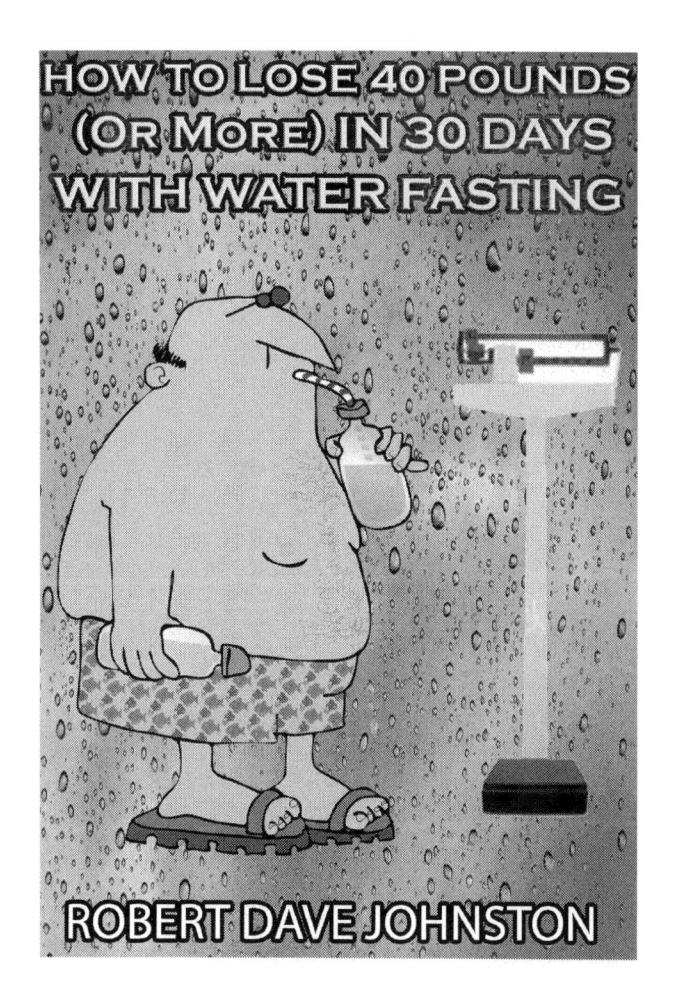

HOW TO LOSE 40 POUNDS (OR MORE) IN 30 DAYS WITH WATER FASTING

ROBERT DAVE JOHNSTON

Introduction

Welcome to **How to Lose 40 Pounds (Or More) in 30 Days with Water Fasting**. This is the book that I've been wanting to write for a long time. Why? Because water fasting transformed my life more than 10 years ago. If you've read any of my other books, then you know the sob story. I was obese and trapped in a destructive cycle of binge eating.

I had lost all hope for a better life and locked myself in a trash-filled apartment to eat myself to death. It was at that dark moment that I first thought of fasting. Out of nowhere, the idea came to me that I had to stop eating for 30 days so my mind, body and spirit could detox and heal. I had vaguely heard of water fasting in the past, but it wasn't anything that I was intimately familiar with.

In desperation, I threw away the last of the pizza and beer; I began to fast. Things did not go very well. Six hours later, I was stricken with intense hunger, nausea and headaches. Fear and rage weren't too far behind. Needless to say, the acute physical and mental symptoms took me down for the count; two hours later I was at the nearest donut shop gorging (*medicating*).

I had tried to diet many times and always ended up binging. So this latest debacle was really nothing new. But something **WAS** different. I was intrigued by the cavalcade of symptoms that had emerged. Having worked as a writer and researcher, I was filled with a million questions about fasting. I remember thinking: "*I have only not eaten in a few hours. Why am I feeling so physically and emotionally sick? What in the world is going on?*" I felt like the drug addict who ran out of dope and had gone into withdrawal. "What?" I said aloud. "Could fasting have incited some kind of withdrawal? But why? How is that possible?"

I became a man on a mission. I devoured countless books on fasting, both religious and secular. I wanted to know what happens to the body when one fasts. This learning process took me to writers, librarians, priests, holistic doctors, vegans, atheists, agnostics, witch doctors, Indian medicine men and, last but certainly not least, a fringe group of *'life-extensioners'* (*people who subscribe to the tenet that the less one eats, the longer one will live*). I personally believe in life extension through calorie restriction, but some of those people were gaunt, sickly and carried a message that, in my opinion, was extreme and harmful. I remember telling one of them: "Buddy, there's a fine line between calorie restriction and anorexia, and you're tap dancing awful high on that tightrope." He just looked at me and gave me a faint smile. That day I learned a very important lesson:

A misused discipline can easily morph into sickness protected by denial and blind fanaticism.

Over a period of 18 months, I gathered volumes of information about water fasting, juice fasting, dry fasting, liquid diet fasting, religious fasting and intermittent fasting. I was like a sponge; what I learned totally blew my mind. The amazing book, **Celebration of Discipline** by *Richard J Foster* has a chapter on fasting that had a profound effect on my mind and heart. When I read it, a rush of clarity covered me from head to toe. I felt that I had found the truth and discovered a solution to my sickness and obesity. What was the truth? It was not very flattering, but I came to realize that I was a **Food Addict**. People had thrown those two words at me many times over the years, but I was never moved. That day, however, scales fell from my eyes; I saw my life with unprecedented clarity. "Robert," I said to myself, "you're a full-blown food addict. You need to do a 30-day water fast to lose weight and purge your body of the trash you've been eating for so many years."

The plan was set. It was all I could do to keep from bursting out in laughter. If a few years prior someone had told me that I was a food addict and needed to fast for 30 days, I would have told them to *screw off*. I would have argued with him or her every step of the way. **Refute, deny... Refute, deny – that was my modus operandi**. But no more. The resistance left me, **I became 100% willing to do whatever it took to lose the weight and restore my health**. I had been smoking one-to-two packs of cigarettes a day for many years. Without even the slightest hesitation, I reached into my pocket, pulled out an almost-new pack and threw it in the trash. I sensed freedom washing over me; it was time to make a brand new start.

I started my first '*official*' water fast around March of 1998. I weighed myself on Day 1 and tipped the scales at 318 pounds. I'm six feet tall, so my ideal weight is 195 to 210 pounds. I needed to lose in excess of 100 pounds! To be honest, I was very scared when I saw those numbers. They seemed to be laughing at me, telling me that I was crazy and that I would never make it. But it **DID** happen.

Rather than 30 days, I water fasted for 40 days. It was very tough for the first two weeks; hunger, nausea, headaches, irritation and sleeplessness assailed me. The mind was constantly inviting me to break the fast and giving me endless reasons why it was better to abort – for now. But I had crossed the line.

I was so sick and tired of being sick and tired that I grit my teeth and walked through the discomfort, drinking lots of water, green tea and seltzer (*sparkling water, club soda*). One day at a time, I did it.

On *Day 40* of the fast, I got on the scale again. I closed my eyes tightly in fear of seeing numbers that would mock my hard work. When I finally peeked with my right eye, the digital scale said that I weighed 258. I had lost 60 pounds in 40 days! To make a long story short, after that fast, several others and the adoption of a structured eating plan (*outlined in this book*), I finally reached my target weight of 195 pounds. I remember falling to my knees and weeping when I saw those numbers on the scale. Being thin: *A dream that I thought I'd never reach but accomplished nonetheless.*

Altogether, it took me 18 months to lose the last 63 pounds. Why so long? Because, rather than fasting and fasting and fasting, I realized that **I needed to adopt a clean and healthy structured diet**. I had to learn how to eat! For decades, I ate whatever I wanted, anytime, anywhere. I could feel the inner resistance and rebellion when my mentor John Benitez talked to me about following a *'structured diet.'* But I was willing to do whatever it took. I had proven to myself (*more than once*) that things never worked out when I was pigheaded and did things my way. I had to learn humility; I had to reach out for help. And the effort has paid off in spades! Today, my weight fluctuates between 195 and 205. Beyond that, **I haven't gained a single ounce back**. Why did I share all of this with you? Because I want you to know that the task at hand, while challenging, is attainable. Let me be blunt: Water fasting for 30 days may very well be the hardest thing that you will do in your life. The question is whether or not you have reached the point of no return. Is losing weight and improving your health the number one priority in your life?

Do you realize that **NOTHING** is more important than this? That your entire life depends on your health? Before I did the first fast, I recall standing in front of the mirror in my underwear; my entire body was covered with thick blubber, my chest was so puffy that it looked like I had breasts. With tears running down my cheeks I yelled: **ENOUGH IS ENOUGH**! That was a crucial moment; it separated my life prior to my life after. Deep inside my soul, **I made the decision that I would lose the weight and recover my health, regardless of the**

discomfort. I didn't care if my body screamed and yelled for pizza, donuts and cheeseburgers; I was going to go all the way and nothing was going to stop me. Let me ask you: Are you there? Do you know in your heart of hearts that this is what you have to do? Are you prepared to do whatever it takes to accomplish your goal? Are you sick and tired of giving in to your appetites and allowing your belly to control you? If you can feel that 'call' inside your heart, then nothing can stop you. You WILL finish the fast. How does one receive that 'call'? By understanding that IF NOTHING HAPPENS, NOTHING HAPPENS.

Millions of people dream about being lean and healthy; they hope and wish, but they refuse to get off the couch and take action. Or maybe they do start some kind of weight loss program; however, the moment hunger (*or any discomfort*) surfaces, they throw in the towel. Since they want weight loss to be easy and painless, they never achieve it. They are petulant, slothful and arrogant; they often believe that things should be easy, and that they **shouldn't have to go through any discomfort**. If any of these behavior or thought patterns describes you, I challenge you to release them and take a firm step forward. If we don't do this now, then when? Tomorrow? Let me tell you something: **There Is No Tomorrow!** Today is the day when your entire life will begin to change for the better. And you won't be alone. I have done many long water fasts and am well aware of the peaks and valleys. Furthermore, as a bonus, you also have access to my **Fasting Masterclass,** a 6-module multimedia presentation on fasting with tons of information, encouragement and inspiration. You'll have .PDF files, MP4's and MP3s, as well as M4Vs for the IPhone and Android. So even while you're going through the fast, no matter where you are, I'll be right next to you! For instructions on how to access this online resource, check the back of this book.

Warning: This book presents instructions on how to carry out and break a prolonged water fast. I strongly encourage you to get some basic blood tests done so that you can gauge your current health condition. Do not disregard any instructions given to you by your doctor in favor of anything that you read here. Do not stop taking any medication without your doctor's approval. If you are experienced at fasting, then you probably are ready to jump in and do the 30 days right away. On the other hand, if you are new to fasting, there is no harm in doing fewer days at first, until you get used to how your body responds. My point is this: **Water fasting is harsh medicine.** If you are unable to fast for 30 days immediately, don't be hard on yourself or give up. Keep trying... give your body time to get used to calorie restriction. Over time, facing hunger, cravings and detox symptoms will give you added mental strength to fast for longer periods of time. This is not a race; rather, it's a long-term marathon that lasts for life. Find your pace and then challenge yourself each time to go a little further. To this end, I recommend my other book **The Intermittent Fasting Weight Loss Formula**. In it, I talk about the intermittent fasting system that I've used for many years to keep myself thin and healthy. Now let's take a look at the plan of action so that you know what to expect as we move forward.

Chapter 1

Plan of Action

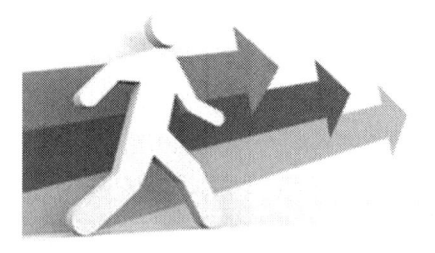

In the first part of this book, we will talk about fasting, what it is, how it works and how much weight it can help you lose. From there we'll look at several fasting studies and how proof continues to mount that calorie restriction can be good for our health. I'll mention some diseases that fasting has been proven to help prevent and even heal.

We'll also see the emotional and spiritual benefits associated with fasting and I'll outline a simple yet powerful way to pray for yourself and others while fasting. Immediately after, we will talk about how much weight you can expect to lose through water fasting, and in how long. Having covered that ground, we will move into the

14-Day Pre-Fasting Phase, during which you'll be asked to clean up your diet so that your body can begin the weight loss and detox process. Cleaning up your diet prior to launching a long-term fast is indispensable because it reduces the intensity of the hunger and detox symptoms. Why? Because during that 14-day period a lot of toxins will be processed out of your body.

Detoxification is basically like going into withdrawal from drugs; the bloodstream and digestive system are cleansed of whatever foods we have been abusing, particularly sugar, fat, alcohol and caffeine. In 14 days, you will have gone through a good part of this withdrawal, so once you start fasting the hunger and other symptoms will usually be milder. In addition, since you will be eating a clean diet, you'll lose anywhere between three to 10 pounds. It is **VERY** encouraging to see the scale go down before you even start fasting!

The 14-Day Pre-Fasting Phase is very powerful because you make progress right away. Furthermore, during these two weeks, you'll start to get a feel for how your body reacts when calories are restricted. A lot of people skip this preparation phase and jump directly into the fast. I discourage you from doing so. Here's a motto that has helped me a lot through the years: **SLOW IS FAST**. I realize that you may be eager to see the pounds drop off of your body. But, in my experience, the more thorough you are in the beginning, the higher the likelihood that you will break the fast appropriately, make permanent eating-habit changes and keep the weight off. People who are overeager and rush the process are prone to making mistakes. All it takes is one impulsive act to blow all of your hard work.

So please remember: *Slow is Fast*! French military leader *Napoleon Bonaparte* was being dressed by his valet prior to a crucial battle. Seeing that the valet was rushing, he looked at him and said: *"Please dress me slowly because I'm in a hurry."* My message is this: Take your time with this process. Follow all of my instructions, even if they seem petty or insignificant. I've been through this, so I am aware of the challenges and nuances. Stick with me and follow my directions to the very best of your ability. After the cleanup phase, we will set the *'mental foundation'* through a series of written exercises that I will ask you to do. You will need a journal to complete our work, so if you don't have one, I implore you to purchase a nice one as soon as you have a chance. Don't get just any old notebook or pad. Get a stylish journal that represents your personality. This journal is going to record your transformation, so we want it to be a very special book that you can go to time and again for many years to come. I have tons of fasting journals and I cherish them all. To look back at what I was thinking and feeling so many years ago, to see the nuggets of wisdom that came out of nowhere...it's something that you definitely do not want to miss.

As part of our *mental foundation* work, I will give you some of my very best tricks and techniques to overcome hunger and detox symptoms so that you can go all the way and accomplish your goals.

Moving along, we will talk about fasting detox symptoms, what each of them means and what you can do to get through them.

From there we will jump directly into the fast. You will have 10 motivational messages to help you through the fast, as well as the audio and/or video recordings from the *masterclass*. I encourage you to download the .mp3's into your favorite player and listen to them throughout the day. Listen to my voice day and night while you are fasting. Listen to my voice until you get sick of it! There are portions on each module specifically designed to provide encouragement and inspiration, so keep listening to those audio recordings. Furthermore, I also encourage you to visit the Forum at *Fitnessthroughfasting.com*, sign up and post regularly. There is a great community of folks there that will be more than happy to answer questions and encourage you while you go through your fast.

The next part of the book will provide detailed instructions on how to break the fast appropriately. I will give you specific menus to follow as well as a list of supplements that we'll need. From there I will present you with highlights of my book **The Permanent Weight Loss Diet**, a very simple regimen that I've followed for more than 10 years; following this structured diet has helped me to keep my weight stable. I know that this is a lot of material. Many people tell me that they read the book all the way through once before starting to do the work. That's a good idea. I want you to move from one phase to the other feeling comfortable with the material. This is an important, life-changing process. Water fasting has the power to transform your life. It certainly did mine. So embrace this awesome work! As you know, many things in life require sacrifice and discomfort. Don't let your mind trap you into thinking that *"nothing will work, that you will never make it; that you are not good or strong enough to lose weight and improve your health."* You **DO** have the power. You have the power of **DECISION**, right here, right now to determine that **YES** - you **ARE** going to give it your all. You are **NOT** going to stop until you lose every last ounce of excess weight and reclaim the optimum health that is rightfully yours! As always, please feel free to write me anytime with questions and or comments. My email address is *webmaster@fitnessthroughfasting.com*

God bless you dear friend. May rich blessings reach you from the four corners of the earth until they overflow and cover your life with prosperity, joy, peace and optimum health!

Chapter 2
How Fasting Works

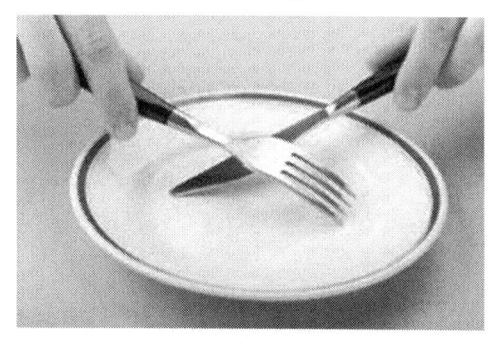

Here I want to talk briefly about the process that fasting kicks into motion, and how the body responds when calories are restricted. The amazing process that I am referring to is known as **ketosis. Ketosis** is the term used to describe the body's response to calorie-restriction. When in ketosis, the body stops acquiring its energy resources from food and begins to *'eat'* stored fat as fuel. Ketosis usually starts after 10-to-16 hours of fasting and/or cleaning up your diet. It may induce a *'flu-like'* sickness known as a <u>Curative or Healing Crisis</u>. We will look at detox symptoms later. The healing crisis is put into motion as the body begins to tap into stored fat for food, causing large amount of accumulated toxins to be released into the bloodstream. This is similar to being vaccinated. If you have received a vaccine, you know that hours later one tends to start feeling a bit under the weather. The reason is that the vaccine fills the body with disease-causing microorganisms; a brief sickness ensues. The same happens when the body goes into ketosis. Toxins stored within fat cells are suddenly let loose. Temporary intoxication results - the *curative crisis*. The body works very hard to expel the toxins through the skin (*perspiration*), urine and feces.

Ketosis continues until the fast is broken as the body devours stored fat for fuel. The healing crisis, however, typically ends after 9-to-14 days, indicating that the body has eliminated all built up toxins. At this time one usually starts to feel stronger and more alert. The healing crisis vanishes and you may feel little or no hunger. Many people tell me that, once they reach this phase, they feel that **they can go on fasting indefinitely**. This is the most pleasant part of the fast. It is like launching a rocket; it initially must penetrate the fierce heat of the planet's atmosphere. If it stays on an upward course, it will eventually get through the atmospheric layer and enter the calmness and silence of outer space. That *'outer space'* experience, I believe, is what ultimate health is all about; it is an experience that we're all entitled to have, **IF** we are willing to pay the price. And I believe that you **ARE** willing; otherwise you wouldn't have bought this book and be reading it now.

How Long Can One Fast?

Most (*healthy and average-sized*) individuals can usually water fast for as long as 50 days before the onset of *'real'* starvation. By the time the healing crisis ends, hunger pangs are reduced and (*in most cases*) become but a minor irritation. Hunger returns (*with a vengeance*) at around day 50 of water fasting (*or more depending on each person's body fat levels*). The return of hunger (*the second hunger as it is referred to*) indicates that the body has consumed all stored fat and has begun to feed on live tissue. This is the start of starvation. The fast **MUST** be broken at once. I experienced this *'second hunger'* years ago when I first started to practice water fasting. It was very scary as I literally felt my skin and muscles being chewed from the inside out. That was my own carelessness. Fasting should <u>never</u> get to that phase.

Eating After Fasting

It's **important for me to emphasize**: While fasting is wonderful and the results can be tremendous, it is **NOT** the fasting in itself that makes the difference. Rather, it is what you do **AFTER** the fast which will determine the **TRUE** benefits that you receive. Fasting for 100 days only to return to eating poorly is a cop-out and not at all what I want to teach you here. I get tons of emails from people wanting to learn about what happens with 40, 60 ... 90-day juice and water fasts. They are interested in quick weight loss, which is fine. However, when I ask them what they intend to do once the fast is over, I either not hear from them again or get a very vague answer like, "*I'll eat better.*"

That type of anemic response tells me that the person has thought a great deal about weight loss, but very little about what he or she intends to do to keep the weight off. **So my message to you is this**: If you are truly serious about losing weight and keeping it off, it is imperative that you realize that **PERMANENT** eating-habit changes are necessary for long-term success. I hate to sound like a broken record, but it is indispensable that you proceed with that fact fixed firmly in your mind. You can lose 40 pounds or more through our work together. But if you do nothing more... if you have not planned ahead as to what your diet will be when the fast ends, then you are setting yourself up for failure. **Let me be blunt**:

Nothing sucks as bad as fasting for 30 days, going through the hunger, detox and sacrifice to lose weight, only to see yourself balloon right back up in a few short weeks after the fast because you didn't change your eating habits.

And I can guarantee you that, if you do not change your eating habits, then chances are **VERY** high that you **WILL** regain the weight within three months. I need you to be very aware of this reality now when we are just getting started. Ponder on what I've just said as we move forward. The good news is that, in this book, I give you detailed instructions on how to follow what I call *The Permanent Weight Loss Diet*. It is a simple, structured diet that, if adopted as a lifestyle, will help to stabilize your weight and heal your relationship with food. **Here's the bottom line**: fasting for weight loss <u>without</u> a plan for permanent eating-habit changes is a waste of time and will <u>**NOT**</u> produce the long-term success that you desire. Lucky for you, you have me in your corner and I will give you all of the information that you will need to lose weight fast and keep it off!

Chapter 3
Fasting Research & Health Benefits

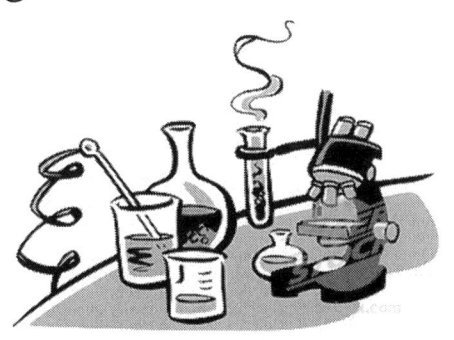

If there is one thing that I'm passionate about, it is reading and studying all of the latest fasting studies that come out. Over the past decade, there's been significant research related to fasting and its health benefits. In this chapter, we're going to take a look at various animal and human trials and their amazing discoveries. If you wish to learn more about these studies, you can find them through a simple web search.

*A recent water fasting study by Joel Fuhrman, MD, Barbara Sarter, PhD, RN, FNP, and David J. Calabro, DC, on fasting and autoimmune disease concluded that, *"Under medical supervision, this therapy is safe and results in only transient side effects. Eating a vegan diet before fasting often* *resulted in partial improvement of symptoms, enabling patients to reduce their medications before the fast. Additional studies of fasting may explain how this treatment induces remission and may clarify our under-standing of the pathophysiology of rheumatoid arthritis and other autoimmune illnesses."*

*The doctors of chiropractic and medicine affiliated with **TrueNorth Health Education Center** concluded in 2001 a 12-year study on *water fasting and a healthy diet* as treatment for various medical conditions, including high blood pressure and diabetes. The paper, entitled *Medically Supervised Water-only Fasting in the Treatment of Hypertension*, says in its brief that, "Our study demonstrated the remarkable effectiveness of water-only fasting in the treatment of the leading contributing cause of morbidity and mortality in industrialized countries."

A second study evaluating the effectiveness of fasting in the treatment of borderline high blood pressure was accepted for publication and appeared in the October 2002 issue of the **Journal of Alternative** and Complementary Medicine.

* A 2011 study reported in **Science Daily** discovered that frequent 24-hour, water-only fasting is good for your health and heart. US research cardiologists indicated that fasting can reduce the likelihood of diabetes and coronary artery disease. Fasting also was found to mend blood cholesterol levels. Furthermore, the study revealed that fasting for 24 hours can boost the human growth hormone that fosters lean muscle mass.

* Another study in the **American Heart Association's Scientific Sessions** (2007) found a link between lower rates of heart disease and people who fast one day each month for religious practices.

* In a paper published **May 17, 2012, scientists** from **Salk's Regulatory Biology Laboratory** found that: *"Mice limited to eating during an 8-hour period are healthier than mice that eat freely throughout the day, regardless of the quality and content of their diet."*

* On April 2011, Utah-based **Intermountain Medical Center**

disseminated the results of their research on fasting, demonstrating that, *"new evidence from cardiac researchers at the Intermountain Medical Center Heart Institute demonstrates that routine periodic fasting is also good for your health, and your heart. Research cardiologists are reporting that fasting not only lowers one's risk of coronary artery disease and diabetes, but also causes significant changes in a person's blood cholesterol levels.*

Both diabetes and elevated cholesterol are known risk factors for coronary heart disease. The discovery expands upon a 2007 Intermountain Healthcare study that revealed an association between fasting and reduced risk of coronary heart disease, the leading cause of death among men and women in America."

Let's take a look at some fasting health benefits in the light of other studies.

Fasting and Autophagy

* A 2010 study by the **Department of Immunology and Microbial Science at The Scripps Research Institute in La Jolla, California** specified that *"short-term*

fasting encourages deep neuronal autophagy." Autophagy (*also known as autophagocytosis or "self-eating"*) is the method by which cells reprocess waste matter and repair. That basically means that, when fasting, the body launches an emergency *'scavenger hunt'* for any nourishment that it can find, consuming everything that it comes across, including fat, toxins, growths and (*in some cases*) even viruses.

Here's a quick analogy: If you were hungry but your refrigerator was empty (*and you had no immediate access to more food*), you would likely open the cupboards and eat what was there (*canned soup and sardines*!).

Once those goods were consumed, you would continue to look for food in different places around the house (*drawers, cabinets etc.*). Such is the process of autophagy.

Being that it fosters the consumption of body-wide toxicity, autophagy is a natural deep-cleansing (*and healing*) machine. I'm not a scientist and certainly that definition isn't all-encompassing. It, however, should give you a good idea of the amazing process that is launched when calories are restricted.

Mark Mattson, chief neuroscientist at the **National Institute on Aging**, has released countless papers over the past decade on the neurological effects of intermittent fasting. In his impressive body of work, it is suggested that, "*IF can protect against brain injury and disease.*" In a 2012 interview, Mattson talked about fasting as it relates to human evolution.

"When resources became scarce, our ancestors would have had to scrounge for food," he said. "Those whose brains responded best – who remembered where promising sources could be found or recalled how to avoid predators — would have been the ones who got the food. Thus a mechanism linking periods of starvation to neural growth would have evolved," added Watson.

Memory Booster

If there is one thing that we all have to face as we get older is increased forgetfulness. Even a teenager can be forgetful. However, cognitive decline does not usually begin until we hit middle age. The good news is that there is growing indication that fasting can give your brain a nice boost as it relates to memory and overall cognitive functions.

Cancer

* In a 1988 animal trial on fasting, forty-eight rats were split up into two groups of twenty-four. **Group A** ate freely for seven days and **Group B** fasted for 24 hours every other day. After a week had passed, both were injected with breast cancer. Nine days after the injections, it was discovered that 16 of the 24 rats that were fasting were still alive. In contrast, 21 of the 24 rodents that were eating had died! Amazing stuff.

* A 2009 human trial brought encouraging results. Ten cancer patients – four with breast cancer, two with prostate cancer, one each with ovarian, lung, uterine, and esophageal cancers – fasted for two-to-four days before and after their chemotherapy. In each case, the harsh symptoms of chemo were consistently reduced. One particular woman in her fifties reported only mild chemotherapy symptoms while fasting. So much so that she actually was able to resume her normal daily activities. When,

however, she did **NOT** fast, the chemo symptoms became very pronounced and uncomfortable.

Chapter 4

More Fasting Health Benefits

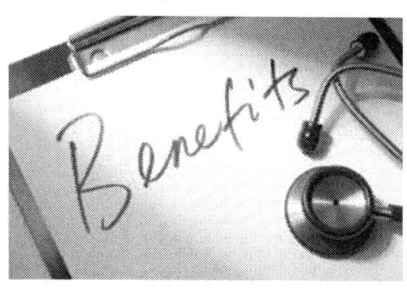

I want to make it very clear that by no means am I saying that everyone should abandon medical treatments and simply start fasting. What I **AM** saying, is that water fasting gives **YOU** a cocked-and-loaded weapon that you can use to take care of your body and health - **IN ADDITION** to conventional treatment. Does that make sense? **PREVENTION** is the key word. The more you do to **PREVENT** illness, the less likely you'll have to rely on traditional medicine to *treat* disease. Why? Because you will be healthy! It's all about balance. I don't talk down about medicine or doctors. I believe in **Personal Empowerment and Responsibility**. It is, after all, **YOUR** life, is it not? Let us look at other conditions that have been improved through the discipline of water fasting.

Cardiovascular & Heart Disease

The benefits of water fasting have become increasingly-evident in chronic cardiovascular disease and congestive heart failure.

* Fasting reduces triglycerides, atheromas, total cholesterol and increases HDL Levels.

Pancreatitis

In one trial of 90 people with severe pancreatitis, water fasting was found to be better than other types of medical treatments. Gastrointestinal medical procedures were **NOT** found to equal the benefits of fasting. In other words, those who fasted were relieved of their condition without the need for any other treatment.

Hypertension

In one clinical trial, 174 people with hypertension water fasted for 11 days. Initial blood pressure in the participants was either in excess of 140 millimeters of mercury (mm HG) systolic or 90 diastolic, or both. Ninety percent of the participants achieved blood pressures of less than 140/90 by the end of the trial. The higher their initial blood pressure, the more their readings dropped. What is your blood pressure, by the way?

Osteoporosis

Fasting induces significant anti-inflammatory actions in the body which result in reduced pain. Fasting also helps the body to produce new bone deposits in areas affected by osteoporosis.

Arthritis

A number of studies have found that fasting is effective for relieving rheumatoid arthritis and osteoarthritis. This is huge considering the terrible pain and disfigurement of limbs that can occur when a person is stricken by this illness. One of my childhood Godfathers went from a charming, amazing poet and singer, to - *years later* - being nearly bedridden by pain because of arthritis. His hands were deformed and he could hardly hold a glass of water. It was a crushing experience to see him in such pain. If you suffer from this condition, water fasting may help.

Other Diseases

Other diseases that have responded to fasting are: neurosis, asthma, irritable bowel syndrome, acne, stomach parasites, fever, hives, various allergies, fibromyalgia, schizophrenia, gout, multiple sclerosis, psoriasis and liver toxicity and/or hepatitis. I suffered from liver toxicity for many years. Today, nearly all symptoms are gone. I know that fasting has a **LOT** to do with the drastic improvement in my health!

Depression?

Is it possible that fasting can help to alleviate and perhaps even cure depression? Based on Watson's findings about fasting and neurologic health, one could possibly say so. I myself have had bouts with severe depression. In 2012, I went through several months of deep-seated sadness and listlessness for no apparent reason. In hopes of finding relief, I launched a long-term water fast. I actually fasted for 50 days, my longest water fast ever. By the time I reached day 21, the depression had greatly diminished. Once the fast was over, the sadness and other symptoms were pretty much gone.

Chapter 5

Is it Safe for Diabetics to Fast?

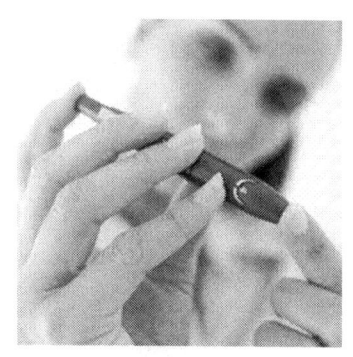

Water fasting has been found effective in the treatment of *Type II Diabetes*, often reversing the condition permanently. Amazing! I wish I would have known about the benefits of water fasting 20 years ago. I would have been able to help my dear grandfather, who died as a result of this terrible condition.

Type II diabetes is becoming a huge problem in the US, now showing up even in children due to obesity. If you are overweight or have notable fat deposits around your midsection, your doctor may want to check you for insulin resistance - also known as *pre-diabetes or impaired fasting glucose IFG*. A fasting glucose or fasting insulin measurement test will determine if your body is producing and properly utilizing insulin. If the test shows signs of trouble with your body's capacity to produce and/or use insulin, then immediate calorie restriction is imperative to drop the dangerous pounds and get your health back on track. Quick weight loss (*and the adoption of a structured and healthy diet*) can notably reduce your risk of developing full-blown diabetes. Even if you have never had a fasting insulin measurement test, you may still be at risk if you're more than 20 pounds overweight. Prompt weight loss and detoxification is indispensable, and little can help you to accomplish that faster (*or more thoroughly*) than water fasting.

I receive frequent emails from diabetic patients asking me very key questions:

* *Is it safe for me to fast?*

* *How long can I fast without being in danger?*

* *Do I still take insulin when I fast? If so, do I take less? How do I know how much?*

* *How will fasting insulin levels change if I don't eat for more than three days?*

The answers to these questions depend on a variety of factors, including age, race, eating habits, general health condition, weight, type of insulin used and metabolism rate, among others. Doctors of holistic medicine that I've spoken to said that juicing is the safest form of fasting for a diabetic. Why? Because, although not eating solid food, the juice continues to provide some caloric intake.

Therefore, the person can keep taking his or her insulin as usual. The dosages, however, may be lower if so indicated by a physician. If a diabetic is going to fast, it should be (*at least initially*) for a short period of time and under medical supervision. If you're a diabetic, by no means should you fast and adjust your insulin dosages arbitrarily.

Diabetics Who Should NOT Fast

But there are definitely some diabetics who, fasting insulin test or not, should not fast for more than a day or two at most (*unless supervised by a doctor*). These include:

* *Diabetics who are not committed to cleaning up their diets and getting more exercise*

* Elderly patients that are weak and lack alertness

* Those with poorly controlled Type I or Type II diabetes

* Diabetics with infections such as acute purulent bronchitis, recurrent chronic bronchitis and bronchiectasis

* Long-time Type I diabetics who are physically deteriorated (eyes, kidneys, heart)

* Diabetics with complications as hypertension or angina

* Persons with a history of diabetic ketoacidosis (high blood glucose levels caused by illness or taking too little insulin)

* Pregnant diabetics

Any diabetic that starts water fasting and has two or more episodes of hypoglycemia and/or hyperglycemia should stop at once and see their physician.

Chapter 6
Emotional & Spiritual Benefits

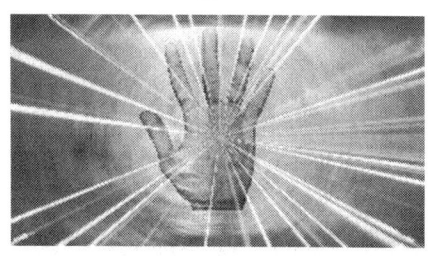

Another powerful benefit of water fasting has to do with inner healing and renewal. Fasting on a regular basis has been the key to my physical and emotional healing. Without fasting, I'd still be plagued with depression, bitterness, fear, isolation, suicidal ideation, hopelessness etc.

Fasting helped me to heal faster because it led me to place greater emphasis on spiritual growth. Fasting put me face-to-face with all of the negativity and emotional pain that tormented me. Being able to face and process this pain has allowed my spirit to grow. Today my job is to remain vigilant and quickly uproot and throw away the mental weeds that try to break the surface. Where there used to be only fear and unbelief, now there's faith and hope.

What I mean is this:

Without fasting, the negative emotions and belief systems controlled my thoughts, emotions and behaviors. They were very painful to resist. My heart and soul were weak and beaten. All I could do was sit in a corner taking blows, *'hoping'* that it would stop. **I had no willingness to fight because I thought that freedom was impossible.**

Fasting changed all of that by giving my spirit a shot of *'spiritual spinach.'* And. like Popeye, I was able to rise and fight against the internal bullies that wanted to keep me down. I experienced a profound physical, mental and spiritual revolution. There is **NOTHING** that can't be transformed, refreshed and/or healed through the spiritual power one gains with fasting.

The answers are within and waiting to be seized. But getting in touch with the spiritual is challenging because we live in a material and superficial world.

*Fasting gives us the opportunity to reconnect with our minds and bodies in a more personal and quiet way

*Fasting increases self-awareness, self-control, self-restraint and patience

We become more attuned to introspection and are thus able to see ourselves with detached objectivity.

*Fasting helps us to "*get out of our own way*"

As the protective layer of the **EGO** yields, we start to feel (*and release*) old memories, thoughts and emotions. This release is crucial because it gives us deeper insight into ourselves. Many have described the process as going into "*the unknown,*" a huge break from their old, established ways of being. During a fast, your body and mind get to unwind from stress. The deeper spiritual dimension, on the other hand, comes alive and is brought to the forefront of our awareness.

As the fast continues, a profound sense of peace and serenity wells up, like a constant meditation is taking place within you. You will feel a fresh and powerful connection with your '*core*' being... the part of you connected directly to the spiritual. This sense of surrender profoundly heightens our spiritual connection. And that connection is the one that has the healing power that we seek. By all means, if you follow a particular religion, fasting is the perfect time during which to seek a deeper awakening. If you wish to explore the spiritual side of water fasting, do this:

1. Take a written inventory of everything *"external and/or physical"* that is going on in your life that you want to see change for the better. This can include health, finances, relationships, or anything else that is troubling you. If there is an ongoing situation that is causing you stress, list it. Be thorough. When you are done, you should have a numbered list with a brief explanation of the negative feelings and/or consequences that each item causes. Then, in another brief sentence, write how you would feel to be free of that situation and how you would use that freedom for the benefit of others.

<u>Example</u>: My binging: a) Causes me great guilt, shame and is harming me physically and keeping me from being more active and social. b) Being healed from binging would give me an amazing sense of freedom and make me a more effective person, both for

my loved ones and others because I would lose weight, be healthier and more alive. **Tip**: Notice that the key in the end is to write *"how being free of the situation will allow you to be of service to others"*.

How would being free of this internal baggage cause you to be more effective for the benefit of others? Example: Being free of these internal chains will cause me to be much more social and open to those who are suffering. I could become a comforter and a motivator instead of someone who is always down and depressed. I could write books about my experience, start a website, etc.

2. Take a written inventory of everything "internal and/or emotional" that you want to change for the better. This often includes character defects that we identify in ourselves such as; shy, lazy, inconsistent, impatient, bitter, angry, depressed, hopeless, resentful etc.

Next to each characteristic, list the negative effect that it is having in your life **AND** write the positive trait you would like to have instead. Conclude this step by writing a few brief sentences on how this emotional liberation would allow you to be a better person for the benefit of others.

Example: My depression: a) keeps me isolated from my friends, I don't want to see or talk to anybody and feel hopeless and dead on the inside. b) I want depression to be replaced with joy. Joy would allow me to see life through laughter and hope and I would be able to comfort others who are hurting by making them laugh or by giving them a lighter perspective on their circumstances.

3) Write a list of specific requests you have related to loved ones or friends that are hurting. Take stock of positive changes that you would like to see come to pass in the lives of the people around you. This can be the healing of a friend that is ill, comfort for a loved-one who is in mourning... anything that you want. There are no restrictions to these requests.

Example: **a)** My uncle: That he would find a job he enjoys and find some financial stability; **b)** My friend John and his wife: That they be able to work out their differences and save their marriage; **c)** My mother: That she be healed of her lower back and shoulder pains and that new opportunities emerge for her to practice her art; d) My wife: That the doors to her profession be re-opened in a quality facility where she is appreciated and loved. **Notice that the request is that our loved ones and friends become better and more effective people.**

4) This is the step where we come to realize our powerlessness. Look at everything that you have written in the first three steps and internalize the fact that you, of yourself, can do **NOTHING** to fix or rectify **ANY** of those items listed. When I first came to that realization, I was floored. You see, I was always the *"saver"*. I always wanted to take care of others and rescue them from their problems. In the meantime, I was dying of a liver illness, was obese, depressed and lived in chronic isolation. I couldn't solve my own problems, let alone the ones of the people around me. Even though we can be intelligent, well-educated and driven – that does **NOT** mean that we are **ALMIGHTY**. This step is designed to give you a **GOD perspective**. Once you are able to admit your powerlessness, then it is time for you to realize that there IS **a Power Greater than Yourself that** CAN **solve** ALL **of the problems you wrote about.**

Here is where a lot of people have problems. They can suspend unbelief for a little while and believe that *'maybe'* there could possibly be a "*Higher Power*" out there. But admit that I am powerless? Never! The problem is that the admission of powerlessness is being viewed as a negative when, in reality, it is a positive. If your car was stuck on a ditch in the middle of nowhere and you had no tools to remove it, what would happen? Do you think that you could use your bare hands to lift the car out of the hole and back on the road?

Or would you need the assistance of somebody else with a truck (*a higher power*) to pull it out? If you sat there day and night refusing to call a truck because that meant you were a loser, would it make any sense? Of course not. Rather, you would admit that you cannot do it on your own and immediately seek for the solution to your problem "*outside of yourself.*" That is what this step is all about. You want to get to a better place in your life. You have goals, petitions and desires that you have put in writing. Now I am asking you to admit that the solution is not within you. However, by looking to that Power Greater than Yourself (*the truck*), you **CAN** find a solution and accomplish your objective.

5) The day **BEFORE** you start the fast, present everything you wrote about in prayer to the God of your understanding. Do it with the internal attitude that **ONLY HE** can remove these problems. Read the list out loud one by one and ask for help. Literally **GIVE ALL OF THEM** to God as you understand Him. Leave nothing out. Place as much emotion as you can behind the prayer. If you have to scream and yell, so be it. *I recall falling on my knees and asking desperately for help as I pounded the wooden floor with my fists and the palms of my hands. I was beaten, hopeless and in dire need of help.*

And so you, too, have admitted your powerlessness and are in urgent need of supernatural intervention, right? God, in reality, becomes your ONLY hope at this point. Ask God for protection while you are fasting. **Spiritual Warfare can be very**

real. Ask God to shield you against all evil, darkness and confusion... and ask for the strength to complete the fast. **YOU ARE READY!**

Prayer for Help

Keep the list with you during the fast and add to it as new requests come up. Spend as much time in prayer as you can. This does not necessarily have to be on your knees. If your religious beliefs call for kneeling to pray, by all means do so. I personally believe in kneeling because it reminds me that **I AM NOT ALMIGHTY** and that there is **ONE GREATER** than me. **But do not let yourself be confused or discouraged by religion or dogma**. This is a very personal moment between you and the God of your understanding. Prayer is simply an act of having a conversation with God. You can pray out loud, in your mind or with others. You can pray on your knees, standing up, lying down or standing on your head. God hears you no matter what. If you are new to spirituality, just keep it simple. One does not have to utter fancy words or extremely long prayers in order to be heard. A simple prayer is just as powerful as any other if it is done with true desire and honesty. **What I want you to understand is this**: When we pray, we are penetrating the invisible world of the Spirit which is *"more real"* than the material world. I'll explain: Look at an object in the room where you are right now, like a chair. **Do you see it**? Ok. Where did that chair come from? **Did it not first exist in a person's mind?** Yes, it was first invisible, THEN its inventor drew it on paper, then he or she constructed it and – voila! - It is now part of our reality for one to see and touch. So, while fasting, we are focusing our vision on the invisible world. In prayer, we are entering THAT realm and receiving supernatural nourishment, healing, comfort and power. Then we are bringing all of those great gifts back to THIS world.

Spiritual Machine Gun

We are spiritual treasure hunters. And this treasure is freely-given so that we can share it with others. The more we share, the more treasure we receive. This is frequently referred to the law of Karma. **A question I am asked regularly is**: What is the difference between praying versus praying

AND fasting? Big difference. When we pray but are NOT fasting, we are entering the spirit world with a suitcase to place our blessings. With fasting, we enter with a super-sized vault! Or, in terms of overcoming addictions and bondage, prayer without fasting gives us a hammer to fight the enemy. With prayer AND fasting, we receive a machine gun! See the difference? This does NOT mean, however, that to get powerful results or be heard by God one MUST fast. **But there are times in our lives when circumstances call for fasting as a means of adding high-octane fuel to our prayers.** When you have time, you can go to **Spiritual Fasting** at our website and read more on this topic.

If you practice a particular religion, continue to do so. Attend those services as you are accustomed to. In addition to prayer, spend time reading spiritual and inspirational books. Important: Carry your fasting journal with you and write regularly about how you are feeling and what is on your mind. You will be surprised how many times the answers we are looking for come as we write! **Remember also that God**

Uses People. That is often how he talks to us. What I mean is this: Do **NOT** restrict yourself by thinking that the answers to your prayers can only come through a *"burning bush"* or some other type of supernatural occurrence. While these can and do happen, **I have found that most of us receive our spiritual breakthrough in very subtle ways, often involving others**. So be very sensitive to what is going on around you and do NOT place limits to **HOW God can work things to your benefit**.

In 2004 I did a 21-day water fast at another men's rehabilitation center where I was working as a volunteer. I was sitting on a bench outside of the cafeteria. Directly in front of me were these beautiful flowers of different colors: red, yellow, green and blue. I remember sitting there and staring at the flowers intently. "Dear God," I prayed. "If you are with me, please break off one of these flowers. Let me see your power." I was going through a spiritual low and felt abandoned by God. "Pease break off one of these flowers," I continued. "Show me that you're here with me God; that you really do care and listen." Out of nowhere, my friend

Brian came and sat next to me. Seeing my long face, he went ahead and broke off one of the flowers and handed it to me! "It looks like you need a flower to cheer you up," he said with a bright smile. Needless to say, I was blown away. Was it a coincidence? Maybe... or then again, maybe not.

Chapter 7

Fasting and Weight Loss

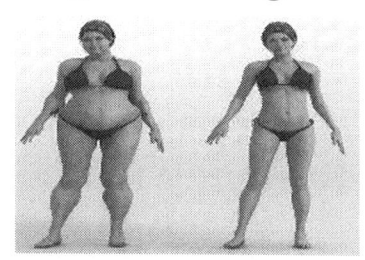

Weight loss while water fasting usually ranges from 1 to 20 pounds (*or more*) in the first seven days. After that, the body (*commonly*) settles into a fat-burning '*pace*' of **one-to-three pounds per day**. Specific weight loss figures will depend on how the body responds, as well as a person's overall state of health. Twenty to 30% of the initial weight lost is comprised of water, not fat.

However, once the early detox process ends (*usually between days 9 or 11*), the body will begin to eat one-to-three pounds of body fat every 24 hours. When I did my first 40-day water fast years ago, I was obese, highly toxic (*from constant binging*) and suffered from a condition called Fatty Liver. I was a complete mess in every sense of the word. During that fast, I ended up losing a massive

60 pounds. I know this gentleman that did a 40-day water fast and lost 75 pounds. The numbers fluctuate from person to person. Still, the results never cease to be anything but extraordinary. In a worst case scenario, you will lose one pound daily with water fasting. But I'm pretty sure that you will lose more. I have coached numerous people through long periods of fasting. On the average, everybody who fasted for 30 days lost a minimum of 40 to 50 pounds. That's why I called this book **How to Lose 40 Pounds (Or More) in 30 Days with Water Fasting**. The title is based on my experience as a fasting coach as well as with my own water fasting efforts.

Light Exercise

A good technique to maximize weight loss while fasting is to include some "*light exercise*" daily for at least half-an-hour. When I say light, I MEAN light. Something like walking, swimming or slow, long-distance bike riding would be good. Stretching is great because it releases toxins trapped throughout the body, facilitating weight loss and expediting detoxification. If you are into weight training, **keep the**

weight light please. The exercise should be comfortable and easy. **DO NOT** have a hard workout while you're fasting! It is dangerous and can cause fainting. A nice 30-minute stroll, swim or light weight training routine will more than suffice.

Try this:

* The first week of fasting, do no exercise at all. Weigh yourself on the seventh day to record your progress. Divide the amount of weight you lost by seven to see how many *'pounds per-day'* you're losing.

* The second week, add a 30-minute daily stroll or swim to your activities. On the seventh day, get on the scale and write down how much weight you shed. Divide the number by seven to determine how many *'pounds-per-day'* you lost. I never cease to be amazed when I see that a simple daily stroll or swim has helped me to lose (*on an average*) 5-to-10 pounds more than the previous week (*when I didn't exercise*). Again, the key is **LIGHT EXERCISE**. If you see that you are getting dizzy and/or nauseous, stop. I'll get more into fasting symptoms later, but weakness, dizziness and fainting **CAN** happen and could result in injury. So please be careful and take it easy. This is no time to break any records or expect your body to function at the same levels that you're accustomed to.

Other Types of Fasting

Absolute Fasting. (*Also known as dry fasting*) is the hardest and strictest form of fasting. It entails going a period of time (*no more than 72 hours are recommended*) without eating **OR** drinking liquids of any kind. There are two kinds of absolute fasts: *soft and dry*. Soft dry fasting allows 'external' contact with water as taking a shower, going swimming etc. With <u>hard</u> dry fasting, the practitioner abstains from **ALL** contact with water, even showering. Dry fasting produces the fastest and most dramatic weight loss, approximately 20 pounds in three days. Most of the weight loss, however, is comprised of water weight because the body goes into dehydration. Although there aren't many studies about dry fasting, it is often used by bodybuilders before a competition to maximize muscle definition. There are some who maintain that absolute fasting could cure the common cold if practiced when symptoms first emerge. I have read cases of people who have done an absolute fast for three-to-five days and were reportedly cured of life-long allergic reactions and conditions. The process behind the healing power of dry fasting is that, since the body is not receiving food or hydration, overall functions are reduced to a minimum. Consequently, it is believed, the immune system has a much greater amount of resources to seek and destroy all sort of sickness - even viruses.

While with juice and water fasting bodily functions slow down considerably, a dry fast reduces them much further. This deeper reduction in body functions, it is believed, gives the immune system ultra-healing capacity. Sort of like having been stuck in a traffic jam and then, suddenly, having the entire interstate all to yourself. You don't have to share the highway any longer.

Therefore, you can step on the gas pedal freely because the traffic with which you were sharing the road is no longer there. I completed a 72-hour dry fast some years ago and can tell you that it is probably among the hardest things I've ever done. You can read more about my dry fasting experience at the main website **FitnessThroughFasting.com**. Dry fasting is dangerous and should not be practiced unless one is **VERY** experienced in fasting and calorie restriction.

Juice Fasting, the most popular of the fasting disciplines, is a time during which one ingests only water as well as the juice from liquefied fruits and vegetables. Juice fasting isn't as harsh as water or dry fasting. Rather than relying only on water, it pumps the body full of amazing nutrients. Overall, 10 days of juice fasting will produce five to 15 pounds of weight loss (*depending on health and body makeup*). Then the weight loss settles on one-to-two pounds per day (*one pound per day is the most common*). One (*obese*) gentleman I worked with some years ago actually lost 75 pounds during a 30-day juice fast. For more on this topic, I invite you to read my book **How to Lose 30 Pounds (Or More) in 30 Days with Juice Fasting.**

Chapter 8

Cleaning Up Your Act

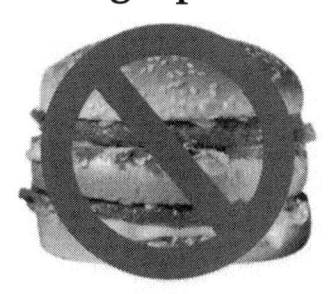

One of the most important steps you can take prior to fasting is to cleanup your act. That means removing all junk from your diet at least 14 days before starting. As I mentioned earlier, this cleanup is very important because it kicks in the weight loss and detox process in advance.

Besides, giving up junk food sends a loud and clear message to your mind that this is <u>not</u> going to be a temporary patch. Instead, I want this to be your first step towards permanent eating-habit changes. Pick the day in which you will begin the entire process. I would suggest that you go through this book several times until you are fairly comfortable with the material and structure. Once you are prepared to get going, pick a day to start the **Pre-Fasting**

14-Day Phase. Starting on that day, cut out the foods listed below from your diet. In fact, cut them out completely - <u>whether or not you're fasting</u>. A lot of these foods may have a strong hold on you. Letting them go in itself will be a big accomplishment. Trust me. Following these directions will give you huge (*and very fast*) results. It may be uncomfortable at the beginning, but you will get used to it. **And you'll be very happy when you see the pounds start to disappear from your body**. For your daily meals, follow the instructions on the next chapter. Right now, let's take a look at the foods that I want you to eliminate ASAP:

Banned Foods

(*Avoid at all times, regardless of whether you're fasting or not*)

*Salt
*Sugar
*Fried Foods
*Cheese
*Dairy Products (*only 'Skim' milk*)
*Red Meat
*Alcohol
*Butter or Margarine

*Fruit Juices (*except for fruit and veggie juices extracted with a juicer*)
*Regular Ketchup (*except low sodium*)
*Junk Food of <u>ANY</u> Kind (*cheeseburgers, pizza, donuts, pastries, cakes, candy etc.*)

The Salt Factor

Cutting out salt was one of the steps which helped me to lose lots of weight quickly, especially in the first few weeks. When we are overweight, a lot of the weight is from water retained due to the excessive consumption of sodium. If you take a look at most of the canned and pre-packaged products sold in supermarkets, the majority of them are packed with sodium. Take a look and you'll see what I mean. All of that excess sodium doesn't do the body any good and it certainly doesn't support weight loss. In the majority of cases, adding salt to what we eat is simply not necessary.

In fact, I no longer add salt to anything. At first it was hard because I had become so accustomed to eating salty. Today, however, I do not add any salt to the food that I eat. If you look at the shopping list I have provided below, you will see that I have listed *'no salt'* seasoning options. So the point isn't to eat bland food that tastes like cardboard; rather, it's to remove that which is excessive and that the body can acquire naturally from a clean diet.

The Sugar Monster

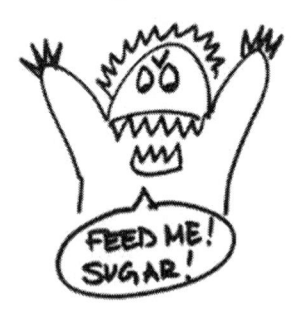

This is the biggie. Most people who are overweight are hopelessly addicted to sugar. I know that I was. I was amazed to learn that refined sugar is actually toxic to the body. If you have ever overindulged in refined sugar and woken up the following morning feeling like a zombie, then you know exactly what I'm talking about. Refined sugar gives us a short-term shot of energy. However, the energy surge quickly results in a *'crash.'* The crash is evident by the ongoing craving for more and more sugar. For people who eat a lot of sugar, these cravings can be very strong - nearly blinding. Sugar gives us that little bit of energy, but it promptly takes it away and - *soon* - we are back to square one - zapped. We never receive the substantial, healthy and lasting energy that we get through complex carbohydrates and lean proteins. So, if you are a sugar addict as I was, I beseech you to fight, fight... fight to overcome this destructive monster! If you do that alone, you will take large strides toward measurable weight loss and health improvement.

I was stuck in sugar addiction for many years. Every time that the cravings hit me, I gave in by eating more refined sugar. The first time that I started to resist, the detox symptoms were so strong that I almost passed out.

I felt like someone coming off hard drugs like cocaine or heroin. Such is the destructive power of refined sugar. Even though it was hard, about 72 hour later, when the sugar was totally out of my body, I started to feel a sense of tranquility and wellbeing that is indescribable.

The cravings were greatly reduced. I realized that the worst was over. As long as I did not fall back into its grasp, I was free of the sugar monster. It was a great feeling; I hope that you, too, get a chance to experience that same freedom.

My point is this: No matter what the short-term discomfort may be, letting go of refined sugars is **the very best thing I have ever done for my physical and mental health**. I say *'mental health'* because sugar caused me to always be in a state of confusion, depression and anxiety; it curtailed my ability to function.

In addition, I kept waking up in the middle of the night craving more, more and more sugar. My sleep patterns were chaotic. Can you relate to any of these symptoms? **Do not compare**. <u>Identify</u>.

Even if the symptoms you experience *'aren't as severe,'* as mine were, you still will do yourself a huge favor by eliminating refined sugar. This is the beginning of the process.

Let's take a look at the typical shopping list that I fill for my pre-fasting cleanup diets. Then we'll dive directly into sample menus that you can follow during the two-week pre-fasting preparation (*and after the fast!*)

Shopping List

*****Boneless Chicken Breast**
*****Extra Lean Ground Turkey Breast** (*no deli turkey*)
*****Egg Whites** - I use the liquid egg whites that come in a box because all I have to do is toss them in the pan. Besides, I always make a huge mess separating the yolk!
Low Sodium Tuna Fish - This kind usually can be found in envelopes rather than cans.
*****Fresh Fish** (*Tilapia and Grouper*)
***** Salmon** (*Once Weekly ONLY*)
*****Baked Potatoes**
*****Sweet Potatoes**
*****Quaker Oats** (*Whole Grain, Quick Oats*)
*****Cream of Wheat** (*White Box*)
*****Cream of Rice**
*****Pasta** (*Whole Grain or Whole Wheat - No Egg Noodles*)
*****Brown Rice** - I am lazy and use the boil-in-the-bag rice.
*****Fresh Green Vegetables** (*Broccoli, Carrots, Cauliflower* etc.) - These are great for steaming. I usually purchase the bags that come with them already pre-mixed. You will find a lot of different veggie combinations to choose from in these pre-mixed bag selections. I like them because all

I have to do is wash and steam them.

Balsamic Vinegar

Garlic Powder

Onion Powder

Enrico's No Salt-No Fat Spaghetti Sauce (*Or any other no-salt brand that you can find*)
This Enrico's brand may be hard to find. Check out the *'health food'* area in your supermarket or a separate shelf in the pasta aisle with the healthy pastas and sauces.

Stevia Sweetener (*Not Equal or Splenda*) Stevia is a leaf and is not piled with all of the chemical trash they put in other artificial sweeteners. It does have a bit of an aftertaste, but you will get used to it after a while.

Any Sugar-Free and Low-Sodium Salad Dressing - It may take a few minutes to find the right salad dressing that meets these parameters. Ask the supermarket clerk for assistance if you are unable to see anything in the shelves. My personal favorite is the *Olde Cape Cod Raspberry Light* dressing.

Mrs. Dash No Salt All-Purpose Seasoning

This shopping list is part of the **Permanent Weight Loss Diet** that I will describe in detail as part of your *post-fasting process*. So it is good that you start practicing now with the menus and food choices. Once our work is completed, I want you to continue following this diet on your own. Make a commitment to follow it for at least one year.

You will be amazed at the results. Not only will you not regain any of the weight that you lost, but your digestive system will be clean and healthy. You will feel better mentally, physically and even spiritually. For people like us who were very overweight and ate poorly (*or destructively*), it is very important to adopt a structured eating plan so that we can establish order in our eating habits and develop a healthy relationship with food.

Rather than using food as a drug to *'get high,'* and receive immediate gratification, we come to view food as the sacred substance that nourishes, strengthens and heals our bodies and sustains our very lives. I would not dare gorge on pizza or donuts today. To me, that kind of debauchery would be disrespectful to my body and to the life essence within me. To be sure, following a structured eating plan has restored me to sanity. I no longer behave like a vicious animal binging for days at a time until it felt my stomach was going to burst, then vomiting all over myself so that I could keep on eating. Instead, I am at peace with food and I'm at peace with myself. And that is the outcome that I want for you as well. If you are willing to follow my instructions, there's no reason why you cannot get there in the coming weeks and months.

Chapter 9

Eat Six Times Daily

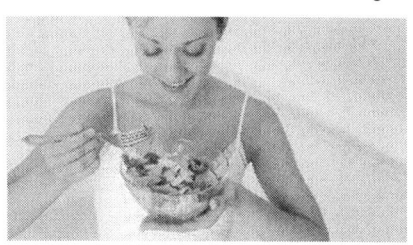

Eating smaller meals with greater frequency, totaling six meals per day, is one of the strategies that will help you to receive the most benefit from this program. So I want you to observe the banned foods list, as well as change your eating structure to one of six smaller meals. This method will <u>accelerate your metabolism</u>, meaning that the body can process and eject toxins faster and with greater efficiency. The metabolism is like a fire.

Let me give you an analogy to illustrate. Imagine that you were stranded in a very cold place and need to keep a fire burning to survive the night. Would you be better off dumping a huge amount of firewood at once, or would the fire burn longer and keep you warmer if you added small amounts of wood frequently? Of course, the answer is the latter. The more frequently you eat (*observing the banned foods list*), the better you will feel and the more energy you will have. Consequently, the metabolism will work evenly and continuously, which results in faster weight loss and elimination of toxins.

Having larger meals with less frequency is like dumping a large amount of wood into the fire. You will get one heck of blaze initially, but it will die out sooner and not provide as much heat (*energy*) as it would if you had added the wood more sparingly. This is what causes the monster cravings that keep people trapped in binging and overeating for years. If you want to disconnect the cravings and succeed in detox cleansing, eat more frequently.

Please note: **The diet adjustment doesn't have to be hard**. Six meals per day include breakfast, mid-morning snack, lunch, mid-afternoon snack, dinner and evening snack. So this is not a *starvation* diet by any means; you can still eat generously while also meeting your detoxification goals. The key is *quality of food,* and that's what this diet emphasizes. To help you see how this works, here is a sample menu from a typical day in my life:

Sample Menu

Breakfast 8:00 AM

1 Cup of Oatmeal with 1 Cup Skim Milk, a Handful of Raisins or Plums

Three Egg Whites mixed with, 3 OZ Ground Turkey

1 Cup of Green Tea with Stevia

Mid-Morning Snack 10AM

1 Apple or Pear Mixed With One Cup of Nonfat Yogurt (*Plain*)

OR, **ONE** Apple, Pear, Banana or Other Fruit

Lunch - Noon

Big salad with lettuce, tomato and other veggies you may like. For dressing, use olive oil (*no more than 1 teaspoon*) and balsamic vinegar.

1 Envelope of Low-Sodium Tuna

1 4OZ Baked Potato or Sweet Potato

Mid-Afternoon Snack 3PM

Same as before - I usually have a piece of

fruit mixed with non-fat, plain yogurt. At this time in the afternoon, I also drink another cup of green tea. As we saw earlier, green tea has energy-boosting and body-heating properties. It will help to give you a pep as well as calm hunger pangs. In addition to green tea, seltzer water (*sparkling water/club soda*) is great to navigate hunger.

Dinner - 6PM

Six-to-eight ounces of chicken, fish or ground turkey (*I like to make turkey patties*)

Large salad as the one eaten for lunch

Steamed Broccoli, Cauliflower and Carrots (*most supermarkets have prepackaged vegetable combinations that are ready to steam and eat*).

4OZ Baked Potato or Sweet Potato **OR** 4OZ of Whole Wheat or Whole Grain Pasta **OR** 4 OZ of Brown Rice

Evening Snack - 8PM

Big salad with 3OZ Chicken, Fish or Ground Turkey - **No Carbohydrates**.

A piece of fruit with Non-fat Yogurt

Cup of Chamomile Tea - Chamomile tea is great to drink at night because it will help soothe hunger as well as calm you and get you ready for bed.

You shouldn't eat anything at least two hours prior to turning in. Sometimes I take one 500 mg tablet of Tryptophan at night to help me sleep. Tryptophan is an awesome amino acid that helps to stabilize mood. At this point I'm done eating for the day and drink only water until 8AM the following morning.

Again -> **Never Eat for the Last Two hours Before Going to Bed!** Do you eat a large portion of your daily calories at night, right before bedtime? When your body is at rest, all of your metabolic processes slow down, you don't burn as many calories as you would while you are actively moving around. When you eat large portions of food shortly before you go to bed, most of those calories will be stored as fat. Unfortunately, some people eat very few calories during the day but gorge at night with a large dinner and snacks. Throughout the day they may have ingested 500 to 700 calories, but close to bedtime they turn around and consume a whopping 2,000 to 3,000 more! Bad idea. Tape your mouth shut if you have to. But eat no more!

Chapter 10
Fasting Detox Symptoms

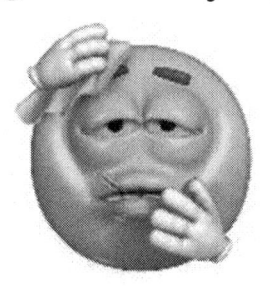

Approximately three days after you cut out the junk and begin the 14-day preparation phase, your body will start to experience what is known as a healing crisis. A healing crisis is a type of *'temporary sickness'* comprised of a variety of symptoms that arise while the body is purging food addictions and excreting toxins through the skin, saliva, urine and feces. In other words, you will be going through withdrawal just like coming off of drugs, nicotine or alcohol. Perhaps your addiction to food has been chronic like mine was, or maybe you just eat too much and lack self-control. Whatever the case may be, if you regularly ate sugar, fatty foods and salt, then going through withdrawal is inevitable. It is important to emphasize that the symptoms experienced are **NOT** an indication that one is getting worse. On the contrary, the presence of a healing crisis indicates that the body is **HEALING**. Hence the name *'healing crisis,'* although it is sometimes also called *'curative crisis.'* The flu-like sickness can last as long as 21 days. However, the worst of the symptoms usually pass within nine days. These are approximates of course. The initial detox process can be shorter or longer depending on the person's body makeup and overall state of health. Ok, **THESE** are the symptoms that stand between you and your cherished weight loss goals. If you can bear these discomforts and annoyances, then absolutely **nothing will be able to stop you.**

Headaches – This one is especially marked for coffee drinkers, but is also the case for persons who consume large amounts of sugar and alcohol. This symptom can really take a person out of commission. If it gets really bad and you need to take a couple of ibuprofen tablets to ease the pain, then so be it. Two, 200 mg tablets will usually do the trick. Don't take more than four in any given day. Coffee will not be in the list of banned foods. However, caffeine is a stimulant and a drug. Cut down as much as possible. A morning cup of coffee is fine. Three, four, five, six more cups during the day is unacceptable. You will become jittery and be more vulnerable to mood swings and impulsive behavior (*more about that shortly*). The good news is that headaches rarely last more than 72 hours, if that.

Dizziness – The body is not used to being deprived of eating whatever it wants anytime that it wants. So you may experience some dizzy spells, especially during the first 21 days of detoxification. The best solution for dizziness is to move slowly and get as much rest as your daily schedule allows. Take care to get up very slowly from a sitting position. If you get up too fast, you may feel like you are going to faint. Some have fainted. A little dizziness is to be expected. But severe dizziness is rare.

Difficulty Performing Basic Tasks – Since you will be eating notably less, it will take some time for the body to adjust, so you will more than likely feel very weak and may have trouble getting around. If you slow down and work at focusing on the individual tasks you are performing, then you will have no problem overcoming this symptom. It is important, however, for you to realize that your body is going through a transition. So you must move slowly and not try to push yourself too hard. You may not be able to function at the same capacity that you're used to. Fine. Slow down and give the body time to work on your behalf.

Weakness means that you need to be extra careful when walking around, and especially when getting up from a sitting position. Avoid harsh and/or abrupt movements. Move slowly, watch your step closely and always have something that you can hang on to if you suddenly feel like you are fainting. This is good advice. One time I totally hit the deck because I got up to quickly from a chair. I missed the corner of the wall by centimeters, but still hit myself quite hard on the floor. This is about improving our health, not about getting hurt. Please be careful. I mean it. Be careful.

Pulsating Hunger Pains that disappear and then re-emerge throughout the day. For some people, hunger is bad in the morning. But for the vast majority, the **hunger troll**

shows up **mostly at night**. Hunger will always be a part of our lives, and it is our task to master it rather than allow it to enslave us as it **CAN AND WILL** if we let it. In my case, hunger was very strong in the first week to 10 days, and then I found myself getting used to always being *'a little'* hungry. I loved it because I began to feel more alert, energetic, and optimistic. I actually **SLEPT THROUGH THE NIGHT** and woke up feeling terrific. Before cleaning up my act, I constantly woke up at night, usually like a raving lunatic wanting to raid the refrigerator. After a while, all of those terrible symptoms diminished and ultimately vanished. I would go to sleep at *11PM*, close my eyes and, when I opened them, it was *6AM*! For me, this was nothing less than a total miracle. And I felt great... refreshed and ready to go! All of that just from getting used to eating less and being a little hungry. Much better than getting stuffed like a boar as I used to.

Bad Breath, Metallic Taste in Mouth, White Sticky Film on Tongue – These are all good indications that your body is eliminating toxicity. Most of these symptoms pass after nine-to-eleven days.

Bad Breath, I suggest that you get sugarless mints and keep them handy until the process ends.

Metallic Taste in the Mouth usually means that there are excessive (*and toxic*) heavy metals accumulated in your system. I recall during my first water fast tasting constant sulfur and '*steel*' in my mouth for like one week.

White Sticky Film on the Tongue is completely repulsive but necessary. It's just another way for the body to get rid of all of the crap we've been eating. For these symptoms, the best thing you can do is to keep drinking a lot of water. Make sure to brush your teeth regularly. Keep a travel toothbrush with you if you spend a lot of time out. Mouthwash is also helpful.

Diarrhea or Constipation – All of the fecal matter adhered to your colon will either start gushing out in diarrhea or incite short-term constipation. I know that this is disgusting, but it happens. If you have eaten poorly for a long time, or have simply abused sugar or fat, your body may respond to this cleanse by starting to expel all of the toxic filth in this fashion.

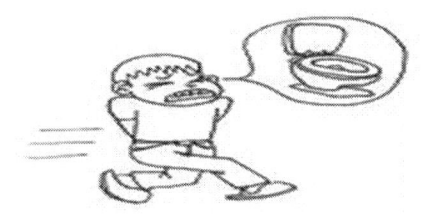

If Diarrhea Strikes, continue to follow the diet and water fast. Should it become severe, see your pharmacist and ask him or her for an over-the-counter recommendation. The clean diet is a shock to the body, but it will finally get the message and react favorably. If you have diarrhea, make sure to keep yourself hydrated. Make it a point to drink at least one gallon of water daily. Stay close to a bathroom at all times. If you go out, make sure that you are always aware where the nearest restroom is. Seriously, you want to get to the toilet promptly anytime you need to.

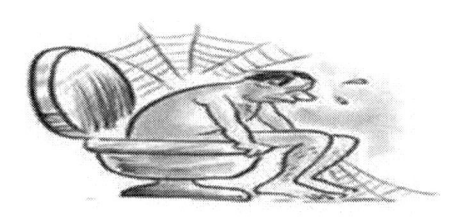

If Constipation is The Case: visit your local pharmacy and ask your pharmacist about a stool softener. I personally use an herbal laxative called **Herbs & Prunes**. It works like a charm every time and is not harsh on my stomach. Take one tablet to start. Do not exceed four tablets in one day. But do this only if you fail to eliminate anything for at least three days. Give your body enough time to do it on its own.

Irritability / Mood Swings – If you have ever seen The Flintstones, you may remember Fred walking around growling on the episode where he is placed on a diet. Be prepared to be a little *short-fused* during this time of heavy-duty preparation. Be aware that you will not be as patient as you normally would be. Tell your loved ones not to take it personally if - initially - you are less social that what they are accustomed. This is normal and will pass! Mood swings also can include boredom, impatience and frustration with the weight loss process. For irritability, it helps to go out for a walk or a bike ride and expel that built-up emotional energy. You can also use the *'delayed reaction'* approach. If something or someone upsets you and you want to lash out, immediately delay your reaction for 30 seconds. I have found that, nine times out of ten, by the time I have counted to 30, I've completely forgotten what I was angry about or simply didn't think it was that important anymore. If the mood swings get really bad, drink a cup of chamomile tea and, if possible, go to bed early. Drink the green tea sparingly until this symptom subsides. Green tea will pep you up and could worsen the mood swings. This emotional see-saw has to do with the detox process, but it is also the body's way of protesting the calorie restriction process.

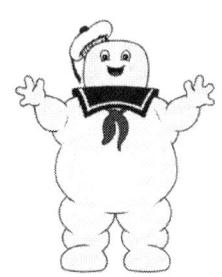

Facial Puffiness & Feeling Bloated – This symptom is much more marked for persons who consume large amounts of salt and/or sugar. The body gets disoriented when sugar and salt intake is minimized. It therefore retains water for some days and becomes *hyper-sensitive* and toxic. I personally was bloated to the max like the *Stay Puft Marshmallow man*. So being puffy was nothing new. It looked like somebody had stuck huge balloons on my cheeks. It was hideous. The diet took care of that and my face today is that of a normal human being rather than a cartoon character.

That's pretty much it. Now tell me: **which of these symptoms is greater than you?** Which of these will you permit to knock you off course? The truth is that <u>NONE</u> of them is bigger or stronger than you. You have what it takes to resist, endure and walk through <u>all</u> of them. And you can accomplish this, <u>WITHOUT</u> having to quit or fall off the wagon. Are you going to *'die'* if you don't eat the junk that the body is asking for? You do not need to *'medicate'* any of your emotions with food. There is nothing to *'fix.'* All you have to do is be still, continue to move forward and wait for the storm to pass. Indeed, you are out of excuses. I n this chapter, I've listed pretty much every challenge that you will experience during the entire cleanup and water fasting process. And, as far as I can see, the only one that can stand in your way now is you. Staying the course **IN SPITE OF** these challenges is the key to success. You have the information. You know what you have to do. The only real choice that you have at this point is to <u>push through and overcome</u>! But you will have lots of gear to help you. Let me show you a few tools of the fasting trade.

Chapter 11
Tools of the Trade

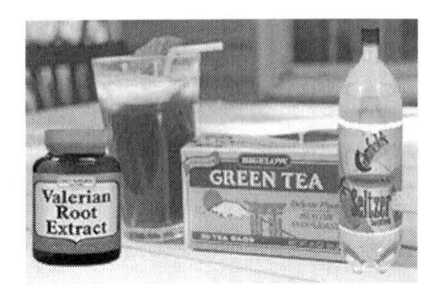

Dealing with hunger and detox symptoms is definitely the primary challenge that we all face when fasting. Over the years, however, I have discovered ways to soothe hunger and minimize discomfort. I'm talking specifically about green tea, seltzer water (*sparkling water/club soda*) and chamomile tea. Let me show you how to use each of these to your advantage.

Green Tea Afternoons

The toughest stretch of time to get through while changing your diet or fasting is usually afternoons. At around 2pm, you may find yourself feeling very hungry, weak, grouchy and just not at all with the program. When this happens, we need to pull out a very special weapon, and that is

green tea. Drinking pure *oolong tea or green tea* extract - *a more concentrated form of oolong tea* - will give you energy and calm physical discomfort. The green tea leaf has large quantities of phytochemical polyphenols called flavonols, commonly known as catchetins. According to a recent green tea study by the Linus Pauling Institute at Oregon State University, green tea fosters weight loss because **the body starts using greater amounts of energy after it is consumed.** This is a direct result of the catchetins' intrinsic fat oxidation and body-heating properties. In short, green tea can help a lot. You can find a good selection at most supermarkets. Have some baggies on you wherever you go so that you can offset that annoying afternoon sinking spell. Be careful not to drink green tea too late in the afternoon. It does have caffeine and may keep you up at night.

The Seltzer Weapon

You should be **constantly drinking water throughout the day.** Any time hunger comes around, fill up an eight-ounce glass of water and drink it down. Have another one for good measure. Every night by 8 or

9pm, you should have consumed as close to a full gallon of water as possible. Yes, you will be urinating <u>**A LOT**</u>, but your kidneys will receive one heck of a detox cleanse. In addition to water, I recommend seltzer water (*sparkling water, club soda*) with a squeeze of lemon or lime. **Seltzer will help to calm hunger pangs and settle the stomach.** Wherever you go, take a small cooler with you packed with ice, drinking water and a few bottles of seltzer. You want to be prepared at all times to deal with any symptoms or hunger pangs that may emerge. Don't overdo it with the seltzer, but drink as many as four bottles daily - especially during the first days when the discomfort is at its peak. And do not drink sodas (*cola*) of any kind, even if it is diet.

In Case of Insomnia

In the first days of the diet cleanup, it is possible that you may have a hard time falling asleep. The reason for this is that the body is releasing large amounts of toxins into the bloodstream and working overtime to heal, cleanse and burn fat. Not being able to sleep can be very annoying, particularly if you have to wake up early in the morning to go to work or fulfill some other obligation. Therefore, if you find tossing and turning, **get up and make yourself a cup of chamomile tea with a squeeze of lemon or lime.** Sorry, no honey or sugar (*use Stevia*). *Chamomile tea* is very soothing and will help you go to sleep. In addition, you can have **one 500 mg tablet of the amino acid Tryptophan**. I use *Tryptophan* all of the time. Together with chamomile tea, it works like a charm and does not leave residual drowsiness when you wake up. As an alternative to Tryptophan, you can take a tablet of *Valerian Root* about half an hour before retiring. In the event that you find yourself still unable to fall asleep, **the best suggestion I can give you is to have a book handy that you can read or, even, go for a short walk around the block.** I took many, many walks during the initial phase of cleanup and found that it helped ease the cravings and relax me so I could fall asleep.

Night Cravings

For some, the biggest challenge is waking up in the middle of the night with monstrous cravings. At this hour, part of the mind is asleep. Hunger may want to take advantage of that and lead you to eat. So you must be cautious and ever vigilant. If you find yourself in this situation, drink a large glass of water and/or have some seltzer with lime. **I like to keep a gallon of water next to my bed so I can grab it immediately.**

<u>Key Tip</u>: **DO NOT** walk to the kitchen!! The kitchen if **OFF LIMITS!** Go to the bathroom, living room or study, but the focus during these night attacks is to <u>NOT</u> go to the kitchen for any reason whatsoever! Have water and/or seltzer close to you – preferably next to your bed on the night table. Yes, the water will probably be warm. <u>DO NOT</u> walk to the kitchen to get ice either! **That is a trick of the mind to get you to open the refrigerator where you will be vulnerable.**

So drink one or two large glasses of water and go back to bed. Repeat this as often as necessary. The wave of cravings may initially come two, three or even four times or more. **OR**, you may not get hit with cravings but, instead, find yourself constantly getting up to urinate. In either case, the result may be that, during those first days, you do not get a great deal of sleep. Hang in there and stick to the instructions. All of this will soon pass and you will start to feel better.

In The Morning

Morning is (*usually*) the most comfortable part of the day. You probably won't feel hunger or any other symptom for several hours. Nothing matches the awesome feeling of waking up, felling light and knowing that you didn't give in to temptation the previous night. Your first task upon arising (*before breakfast*), is to drink **TWO** large glasses of water. You will feel the water going down the belly. It is a great feeling. Drinking water in the morning induces excellent bowel movements which help to expedite the detox process.

Additional Tips: To move your bowels even more (*while you're NOT fasting*), you can squeeze lemon juice into a cup of warm water and add a touch of raw honey with a pinch of rock salt. You can drink one or two cups as soon as you get up. Another alternative is to mix organic lemon juice, warm water, a little maple syrup and a pinch of cayenne pepper. This is similar to the mixture that is used as part of the Master Cleanse diet, a popular fasting detox regimen. If you are having regular and thorough bowel movements on your own, then there really is no need to drink any of these additional concoctions. I give them to you so that you can be aware of the various choices that you have if you start struggling with constipation.

Chapter 12
Setting the Mental Foundation

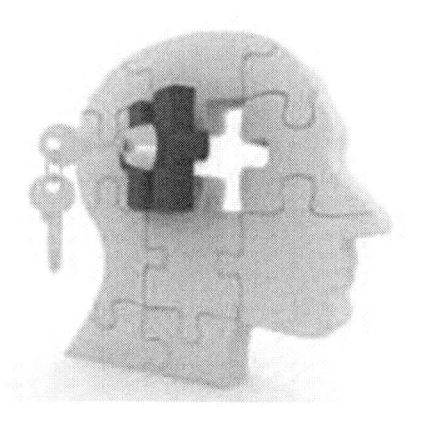

Ok, so you have your list of banned foods, shopping list and sample menus. Furthermore, we have looked at the most common symptoms that you'll likely experience. I've also given you the weapons of seltzer water, *Valerian Root, Tryptophan Chamomile and Green Tea* to help you get through the rough spots.

Now, I want to go even further and present a series of mental techniques and exercises that will give you even more leverage over hunger and detox symptoms. So take out your fasting journal and be prepared to answer a few questions. One of the reasons why people start a weight loss program and fall off is because, when hit by temptation, they are - *at that moment* - unable to remember with sufficient power the important reasons why they want to lose weight in the first place. Blinded by hunger, detox symptoms and other types of temptation, they give in and eat what they shouldn't. The enjoyment, however, is very short-lived as, almost immediately, the **Three Horsemen of Guilt, Shame and Accusation** arrive and start tormenting the person. If you have ever started a weight loss program and quit halfway through, then I am pretty sure that you know what I'm talking about.

The result of this emotional onslaught is that the person often will say "*screw it*" and abandon the diet or fast altogether. "*What's the use? I'm a weakling, a loser... I will never lose all of this weight! Why even try? This is pointless. I'm hopeless!*" Many people are stuck in this demoralizing trap of falling, giving up, gaining weight and then starting the diet again weeks, months (*or years*) later. I can't think of anything that is more frustrating than this. Well, **the questions that I want you to answer here are**

designed to erect a fortress against these ever-lurking foes. Here's my point: If you can overcome the temptation directly when it hits, then you will not put the wrong food in your mouth and start the entire compulsive episode. That's what we want. To stop the *'screw it'* syndrome **BEFORE** it has a chance to take hold. One lady told me:

"Robert if I hadn't eaten that fifth donut, I would be fine." I tried to help her understand: *"It isn't the fifth donut that gets you, it's the first one! If you don't eat the first one, then you certainly won't eat the second, third, fourth or fifth. It is the FIRST one that starts all of the trouble. And it is the first one that we must learn to avoid."* Does that make sense?

So, right now, I want you to take some time and **write the questions listed below in your journal and then answer them with as much honesty as you can muster**. Don't just skimp over them. Take your time and answer them thoroughly and in detail. The answers that you come up with represent the artillery that you will use when temptation invites you to stray from your diet or fast. At that particular moment of temptation, all that will be between you and that piece of junk food will be the answers that you come up with. So here we go:

Anchor Questions

What will happen short-term if I DO NOT resist these urges and continue down the same road? In other words, over the coming days, weeks and months, how is your life going to be and how are you going to feel if you do nothing and allow these habits to go on unbridled? Be as explicit as you can. *(Example: If I do nothing and fail to resist these urges, I will continue to gain weight and feel worse and worse about myself. I will isolate because I'll feel ashamed of my appearance. I won't want to be seen, go out in public. I will be depressed and feel defeated etc.")*

What is the ultimate long-term consequence that I will pay if I do not take action NOW to change these thinking and behavior patterns as they relate to food and eating? Be explicit! *(Example: If I do not take action now and do* *whatever it takes to lose this weight, I will feel like I failed at something that is very important to me, I won't have the same self-esteem because I'll continue to be fat. I will feel defeated and absolutely terrible because there is nothing that I want more than to get rid of this excess weight and look and feel my best etc.)*

What will my life be like in 10 years if I do not take action now? Mentally, physically, socially, spiritually etc... Remember *The Ghost of Christmas Future from A Christmas Carroll*? Well, this is it. Use it! Dig deep into your heart and mind and look at yourself 10, 15 years from now **NOT** having done anything about your weight and health. What do you see? How do you look? How do you feel? How is your health? How is your quality of life? *(Example: Ten years from now I look like a beached whale plumped in the sofa with dark circles around my eyes, no energy to do anything and in deep depression and isolation because I am disgusted with my appearance and have withdrawn from life completely. I am sitting there wishing I was dead etc.")*

Am I willing to pay these negative consequences? Why not? Be detailed. *(Example: because I want to be around for my children, travel abroad, get married, continue to advance in my career, be prosperous, have a lavish life, not develop a chronic illness etc.).* As I said earlier, it is important that you take your time and come up with strong answers. If you just jot down a one-sentence response without giving the questions deep and serious thought, then you are wasting your time. *(Example: I am NOT willing to pay these horrible consequences. I am prepared to do ANYTHING to keep that horrible future from ever coming to pass. That means that I am now willing and prepared to resist any hunger and any temptation so that I can overcome this weight issue once and for all and avoid having to face a future that is so ugly and hopeless etc.)*

These questions are meant to strip your soul bare and **force you to cough up deep-seated thoughts and feelings**. That is not to say that initially you may only come up with one sentence. That is fine. But don't give up... keep meditating on the question and continue to probe your mind and heart for answers. Believe me, they are there!

How would I feel if I STOPPED feeding into these food impulses and began to say NO? (*Example: Empowered, Good about myself, Hopeful etc.*). Why would I feel these positive feelings? (*Example: Because I will have resisted something that harms me, because I will have gained self-esteem, because I would start to feel lighter, healthier, more attractive etc.*). This is the pivotal point where you can begin to see that NOT giving in to these urges is the ONLY way to true happiness and satisfaction. Giving in may feel good at that immediate moment, but saying no and delaying gratification is the road to the ultimate victory that you seek.

What would happen if I resist these urges to eat? Do I feel like I would collapse or die? Can I recognize that these are lies? Explain the reasons the mind gives you as to why resisting these food impulses is *'too hard'* or even *'impossible.'* (*Example: When I am tempted, I feel like I simply cannot resist. The cravings are just too strong etc.*). Can you internalize the reality that this is a lie? That you are **NOT** helpless? That you **CAN** get through it? *(Example: Resisting these cravings is NOT impossible because I will NOT die if I do not give in, etc.).* The key to this question is realizing that any short-term discomfort you may feel from resisting the food urges will pass, that you will not fall to pieces if you hold your ground. As a matter of fact, I can tell you from experience that cravings and temptations rarely last more than 30 minutes. Once they pass, the sense of satisfaction is amazing.

What is the ultimate truth for you? *(Example: I must change my impulsive eating and I must stop giving in to the cravings and food urges because otherwise I will never reach my goal, I will feel unhappy, I will feel unfulfilled, I risk illness etc.).* In view of the answers to all of the previous questions, what conclusion have you reached?

So, to round up, **what real choice do you have than to change?** Continuing to give in to hunger through binging, nibbling and/or compulsive eating is not the answer. It will never be the answer. It will never work. *Continuing to give in to binging,* *nibbling and/or compulsive overeating will always lead you to negative outcomes in your life.* Period. End of story!

Can you admit this to yourself and understand it? Explain why you admit it and why you understand it. If you can admit to yourself that the status-quo doesn't work and that immediate change is imperative, and if you can write in detail the reasons why this is so, then you are on your way to some pretty dramatic changes in your food behaviors.

So this begs the question: **What is your choice going to be?** *(Example: My choice will be to do whatever it takes and go through whatever short-term discomfort I need to in order to overcome and reach my weight loss goals).* Explain the *"why"* of your choice.

What are you willing to do to achieve the life that you deserve? Here we reinforce the previous question with detail of what you are now prepared to do to reach your goals. *(Example: I am willing to walk through the urge to binge, feel the pain of not doing so, deal with hunger pains directly even if I want to give up and give in)* This last answer is important because it provides powerful reasons for you to hang on to when you feel like giving up. So be detailed!

If you follow my instructions and answer the above questions thoroughly and with total honesty, you will have created a <u>very powerful weapon</u> against that *'first bite'* of food that knocks you off your diet, fast etc... Here's how you are going to use these questions: When you start fasting and get hit with hunger, detox symptoms and/or any kind of emotional negativity that makes you want to quit, take out your journal and start reading the questions one-by-one. At that particular moment, try to add more to each one of the answers as you go through them. Focus all of your attention on reading the questions, answers and adding to them.

Give yourself totally to this task.

In my experience, after 10 or 15 minutes, I am re-energized and get a fresh jolt of motivation to continue. The answer of *'how will I feel in 10 years if I don't take action'* is the one that always gets me. The vision of myself ten years into the future still obese and having done nothing filled me with such fear and disgust that I literally didn't care how hungry or weak I got. All I cared about was reaching my goal.

While fasting, you will also want to be in touch with other people that are on the same road. To that end, (*as I've already mentioned*) I put together a *Fasting Forum* where you'll find fellow fasters who are ready to motivate and encourage you. And there are lots of folks there who can use your support as well. You'll be surprised how hunger and detox symptoms often vanish when you focus on giving motivation to somebody else who needs it. Give and you shall receive!

The 5 'D's

Let me share with you the five key steps (*which I call the Five D's*) that helped me to hang on, even when the symptoms and hunger were at their worst. Take your time and put these to practice thoroughly as I know that they will help you. The point of these five steps is to give you the strongest foundation possible for your fast. So don't skip through these or take them lightly please!

DECIDE that you are through with the old

way of things. Resolve in your heart-of-hearts that you **ARE** going to follow through - no matter what. Draw an imaginary line that ends your old way of eating and relating to food, health and wellness, and become <u>totally willing</u> in your inner self to take action.

DEFINE the type of life that you want to have as a result of your new healthy lifestyle. Look at the new activities and relationships you want to engage in. So, as of now, (*if you haven't done so already*) mark that calendar and decide when you intend to start the cleanup and subsequent water fast. If you have truly defined the type of life that you want for yourself, then moving forward with this process is an absolute must. And I'm not talking about tomorrow, next week or next month. I am talking about **RIGHT HERE AND RIGHT NOW!**

DECLARE to your close friends and family that you are through with being overweight and toxic and that you will be implementing some changes during the next months to lose weight and improve your health. Tell them that you will <u>**NO LONGER**</u> be indulging in junk food and that you do not wish for it to be offered. The purpose of this step is to give you some immediate accountability with people that know you. You do not, however, have to disclose your plans to everyone. Disclose it only to immediate family members, people that you trust and that you know won't judge or put banana peels in your path. You may not realize it, but there are some who may actually resent that you are taking hold of your life and health. Be aware and don't let them bring you down!

DESIGNATE a specific person that you trust and tell him or her specifically what you intend to do and why. Ask this person for support during the process and stay accountable to him or her on a regular basis.

Visit the **FitnessThroughFasting.com** forums where you can give and receive lots of support and motivation. There are tons of online forums dedicated to weight loss. Find one that you feel comfortable in and make it a point to get involved with the community. That alone will help you in more ways that you can imagine.

DEVELOP a strong journal where you can

put in writing the reasons why reaching your weight loss goals is important **TO YOU**. Some examples can be; *weight loss, better health, healing from specific illnesses, more energy and vitality, mental clarity, dropping clothing sizes to a particular size, participating in a certain sport, getting married, dating, wearing a bathing suit you always wanted to, having a flat stomach, getting into your high-school-days clothing etc.* These are personal reasons and are crucial because they mean something **TO YOU**... not to your spouse, children or family... but **TO YOU**!

Yes, our loved ones are an immense source of motivation to get us going, but ultimately we have to do this **FOR OURSELVES**. I cannot stress enough the importance of keeping a journal. In it, you can write the dreams and goals that are closest to your heart.

And those dreams and goals will give you immense power to stay the course when you're tempted to give in.

Each time you find yourself weak and wanting to break the fast, you can pick up the journal and read your entries. The more specific and emotional you are when writing, the better. During those moments of weakness, the journal will help you to remember the huge payoff in health and weight loss that you will receive by finishing what you started. Trust me, the immense satisfaction that you will feel when you reach your goal is beyond description; it is a joy and exhilaration that you must experience.

Whatever temporary discomfort you have to go through while fasting is **NOTHING** in comparison to the physical and mental rewards that you will receive. Constantly remind yourself that you want to get this over and done with **NOW**; you do not wish to spend years wishing for weight loss but never achieving it. This is your time. Make it happen!

Chapter 13
Mental Strategies

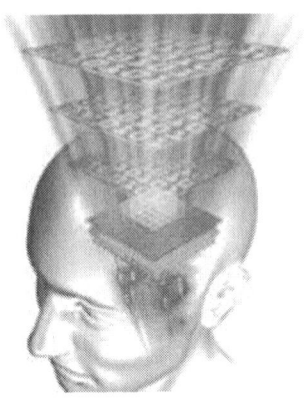

A very powerful antidote to the vicious and crippling cycle of weight loss/weight gain is this: Learning to *"forcefully"* bring the mind to the immediate present when the body, thoughts and emotions beckon you to give up. **It's important to realize that weight loss (and any change in eating habits) will bring most (if not all) of our human weaknesses to the surface.** This can manifest itself in all types of negative and painful emotions, particularly in the first days of a calorie restriction program. You may feel angry one moment, and then find yourself weeping the next. You can go from total and absolute motivation, to wanting to throw in the towel in a matter of minutes.

When one is under this type of assault, the cherished goal of weight loss and improved health can quickly become a <u>secondary</u>, <u>far-away illusion</u>.

At that moment, actually staying the course indefinitely will seem virtually impossible. The mind will attempt to swallow your dreams and trap them in time – all of this fueled by your very thoughts, feelings and cravings. And, to end *the suffering*, the mind will invite you to eat whatever food is in sight – regardless of how toxic and destructive. In fact, the more toxic and destructive the better because *"you will receive more comfort,"* the mind will say. I was struck down by this monster over and over for more than 20 years.

We must expose the enemy in order to effectively stand against it. In this case, the 'enemy' becomes *a warped concept of time that throws our senses (sight, sound, smell) into overload and impulsive (and counterproductive) action.* Ok ... stop for a moment and <u>take a deep breath</u>. That was a lot of information in a few short paragraphs. Are you with me so far? What I have described is **an attack on everything that**

you wish to accomplish. It is the foe in our minds that constantly tries to steal our hopes and dreams! The most baffling part is that the assault is not carried out by an outside force; rather, the prime and sole perpetrator is – OUR MINDS!

In The Present Tense

Much has been written about the power of the present moment. Authors like Eckhart Tolle and his renowned *Power of Now* series illustrate very clearly how our **false perception of time** can cause tremendous emotional hardship and long-term suffering.

My own interpretation of the *present moment* concept is this: Since the past is gone and the future does not exist, any long-term focus on them will usually create anxiety, sadness, anger, fear etc. Why? Because there is absolutely nothing that we can do about the past **OR** the imagined future. The best way to change our future is to live a better present. *We have no power to make time go by faster or to go back in time and relive a past era or moment of our lives.* This is what Tolle refers to as *psychological* *time*. The past and future exist **ONLY** in our minds, nowhere else. They are but illusions and have little *(if anything)* to do with the actual present *(reality)*. A good friend of mine who I will call Paul clearly illustrates how terrible this time trap can be. He suffers from severe binge-eating disorder and, as of the last time we spoke, was 200 pounds overweight. He always starts out strong with his weight loss program, but never lasts more than two weeks. The reason for his chronic relapsing, he says, is that when time starts to pass, he remembers the great times he had in the 1980s and feels an overwhelming urge to *celebrate*. Even though I've tried to *'make him see'* the distortion in which he is caught, the *'celebration'* continues to this day.

The antidote to this crippling *(and unproductive)* state of mind is nothing more and nothing less than **learning to live in the absolute present moment**. Do you know why? Because <u>the present is eternity</u>. And harmful emotions based on the past and future cannot exist in the eternal now. They are gobbled up in the same way that a black hole in space swallows gravity and even light. The present is freedom; and there's no other place to find it except in the here and now. To accomplish this, we must accept the fact that **we are totally powerless over anything else except the present**.

Therefore, wasting time thinking about the past and future will do nothing but continue to contaminate the present. That isn't to say that one cannot reminisce about good times, regress in order to identify and heal wounds, or even plan for the future. Those are all productive ways to live a better *NOW*. However, when the thoughts of the past and future are constant, morbid and not part of any self-improvement effort, then we are *trapped in time* and in danger of acting impulsively as an effort to soothe the emotional pain.

Escaping the 'Time Trap'

I invite you to read this chapter several times until you can identify how this trickery operates in your mind. It may take some time for you to notice it because it often takes place under the level of consciousness. So now, let's look at a mental technique that has helped me to stay the course in moments of intense discomfort and temptation. First of all, when these difficult moments arise and you are tempted to stray from your diet or fast, **STOP!** Bring all of your mental focus to the immediate present. <u>Do this</u>:

*Look at your hands and feet and bring to your attention what you are doing and where you are at that particular time. Are you at the supermarket? At the office? At home? In the car? Are you driving? Walking? Working? Out with friends? Cooking for your family? Example: *"Ok, Robert – you are <u>NOW</u> at the supermarket walking down the cereal aisle."* <u>NOW</u> is the key word.

*Pause and focus your mind solely on what is happening at that moment. When other thoughts and feelings related to food, eating and giving up try to force their way through, push them back and look closely at what is happening around you.

Here's how you can wipe out the craving/desire to break the diet or fast:

*Place Emphasis on Your Sense of

Sound. I wrote this entry in my journal when I was hit by a massive craving for sugar while in a supermarket: *"I am NOW pushing a shopping cart with a squeaky wheel and listening to music playing over the loudspeaker. I can hear myself walking; people are talking all around me; a baby is crying nearby; the cashier is asking for a price check etc."* The key is to listen for any and all sounds within earshot. Go deep. What sounds can you identify that you would normally not hear? Can you hear other people's footsteps? What about the air conditioner or other machinery? Try to discover as many *'new'* sounds as possible. Close your eyes if it helps. Trust me, there are **MANY** things going on around us that we barely ever see or hear. The deeper you go in your search for sound, the quicker the craving will dissolve.

But you can go even further.

Keeping the above two steps active in your mind, **tighten the mental reigns and start to visually peruse everything around you, in detail.** Here's another entry from my journal: *"The floor is gray; the shelves are painted beige; the man in front of* *me is wearing a black pair of pants with a blue sports jacket, argyle socks and two-toned shoes (anybody still dress like this?). I see people coming in and out of the store."* Go deep. Scan your surroundings and focus your sight in as much detail as possible. **Then you can combine both sight and sound and immerse yourself in every little detail that you can hear and see.** It never fails that, within a few minutes, I am feeling better and the craving has vanished. This strategy will require practice, especially if, like me, you have given in easily to hunger in the past. But the more you practice, the deeper you will go and the faster the cravings will disappear.

The Weapons of Sight & Sound

The strategy is to fill your sight and hearing with as much detail as possible of what is happening in the IMMEDIATE PRESENT. At first you may feel silly.

The mind may tell you that you are wasting your time. That it doesn't work. The mind may press you with more acute hunger and/or irritability – you may feel hopeless. It is at that precise moment that you must take the battle directly to the mind and persist with the exercise. If you give yourself <u>COMPLETELY</u> to the technique, you will find yourself – *over a period of 5 to 15 minutes* – immersing your mental energy into **NOW**.

And the <u>NOW</u>, without fail, will <u>ALWAYS</u> consume these attacks! It is guaranteed. There is <u>ZERO</u> opportunity for these imps to survive when the immediate present is summoned.

Lost In Thought

The problem with most of us is that we are lost in our own thoughts and hardly ever stop to look at what is happening around us. I will give you a good example from <u>**MY**</u> own life:

I drove by a flea market daily for three years and <u>**NEVER**</u> noticed it until a friend invited me to visit it. Another time I was trying to find a shoe-repair shop and did not realize there was one a block from my home. I had walked and driven by it constantly, **looking at it but not seeing it**.

Moreover, I lived in a house that was surrounded by beautiful lush trees, many of which were utilized by a variety of birds to breed and nest their young. Most mornings there were countless little birds singing outside my bedroom window. But, honestly, **it is very hard for me to remember ever listening!** If you asked me what the bird song sounded like I would **NOT** be able to tell you! I heard but did not listen.

I spent most of my waking moments trapped in the mind thinking about the past and/or future, barely taking a moment to see or hear the present moment.

Many people live their whole lives in this disempowering state. They are locked inside their own minds, constantly replaying scenarios of the past and future. This elicits unpleasant emotions that, in turn, lead to obsessive and compulsive behavior designed to "*medicate*" the pain. Unfortunately, the obsessive/compulsive action brings only short-term relief. The behavior ends up becoming an overpowering monster capable of consuming a person's entire life via binging, overeating, nibbling, grazing, etc. This mental prison fueled my binging and overeating for many years.

I was always anxious, irritable and

discontent, always reacting to the *lies and distortions* that the mind was feeding me.

In short, the *Time Trap Escape* reminds us to break away from the snare of constant thought. It teaches us to step out of our minds frequently and just **be** by absorbing the sights and sounds of life. The discomfort associated during weight loss is minimized *(and even eliminated)* when one becomes adept at this simple (*yet extremely powerful*) exercise. The soothing calm that comes over the entire body once the attack is over is amazing. It will help you to realize that the demands and loud voices within, ultimately, only have power over your actions <u>if you let them</u>. If you feel daring, I invite you to spend longer and longer periods of time each day in this state of "*present mindedness.*"

The exercise is especially effective while one is fasting and/or making significant dietary changes. It is like doing **mental push-ups.** At first you may only be able to do five pushups, with much struggle and exertion. But, if you continue to train, in a short time you will be able to do more. The same is the case with the mind, my dear friend.

Practicing present moment focus has been my biggest ally. To focus exclusively on what is in front of me. This is difficult because most of us are accustomed to letting the mind wonder aimlessly like a wild horse without a bridle. Weight loss, therefore, goes beyond just eating less and working out. It places us face-to-face with our undisciplined thinking and impulsivity. Calorie restriction disciplines the mind as well as the body. But we must be willing to adopt new thinking strategies that can help us sustain the benefits. *I learned after much trial and error that food was a mere symptom of my undisciplined/obsessive thinking.* Indeed, losing weight will help you to look and feel much better. But the benefits will not last unless you humbly commit yourself to reclaiming control over your mind.

To this end, I invite you to also read my book *How to Lose Weight & Keep it Off by Reprogramming the Subconscious Mind* as well as *The Cravings Ninja Assassin*. Let's look at one more strategy that can help you to overcome hunger and the discomfort of detox symptoms.

Detox Breathing

When tempted to give in, we must pull out every weapon in the arsenal. The *Time Trap Escape* will place you in a position of offense. Now, let's go a step further and continue the counterattack through what I call *Detox Breathing (DB)*. *DB* is one of the most important tools you can use to overcome cravings and temptation. **Breathing is the essence of life**. Without breathing there is no life. I am not talking about the typical *"breathe in, breathe out"* exercise that one associates with meditation or the 1985 movie *The Karate Kid*. That type of breathing is indeed great and I encourage you to practice it.

DB, on the other hand, is comprised of **intense 10-minute breathing sessions designed to give you an immediate physical and mental boost**. I have found this *espresso shot* of oxygen to be amazingly beneficial in reducing mental negativity, hunger and detoxification symptoms. I use it constantly. **The problem is that many people have not learned how to breathe**

properly. They do not realize that reduced oxygen intake causes them to be tired and lethargic; it slows the thought process and breeds <u>depression and negativity</u>.

Indeed, you have tremendous life-giving power in your lungs. One of the first things that I observe when I meet a personal coaching client is the person's breathing pattern. **Nearly 100% breathe shallow**. Very seldom – if ever – do people STOP and *practice the art of breathing*. The moment has come for you to start.

<u>**Special Note**</u>: *Do you snore? If so, you may suffer from a condition known as* **Obstructive Sleep Apnea**. *OSA can make this entire process <u>TWICE</u> as hard because your breathing is blocked while you sleep and the brain does not get enough oxygen. Not to mention that your body cannot fall into the deep sleep required for proper rest. So if you have been blamed for cutting logs and/or roaring like a bear then I encourage you to go see your doctor. He or she may send you for a sleep test to determine if you have this dangerous condition. If so, you may need to incorporate the use of a* **Positive Airway Pressure Machine**. *Weight loss will also*

help.

Detox Breathing in Practice

When a craving or temptation hits, do this: Immediately put to practice the *Time Trap Escape*. Find a place where you can be undisturbed for 10 minutes. Sit down and close your eyes. **Take the deepest breath that your lungs allow**. Breathe in until you cannot take in any more oxygen. Count the seconds as you inhale. Depending on the condition of your lungs, you will be able to count to five or 10. If you are unable to get to five ... don't worry. Your lung capacity will actually improve as you continue to practice *DB*.

Inhale and count simultaneously until your lungs are completely full. As you count, visualize that you are breathing in white, glowing, healing oxygen ... see the white air in your mind's eye. If you are not used to breathing deep, you may feel aches and pains on your back, chest and throat. Those aches will also disappear as you practice.

* Once you have inhaled as much air as the lungs permit, visualize the white, powerful oxygen navigating around your

entire being. Whatever number you reached during the inhalation, multiply it times eight.

If, for example, the inhalation lasted seven seconds, multiply that times eight for a total of 56. Now hold your breath for the resulting amount of seconds, in this case 56 seconds. If you cannot reach the X8 goal, do the very best that you can. Build up to it.

* As you hold your breath, keep visualizing your body being filled with a white light representing the healing oxygen that you inhaled. Observe as the white light covers your legs, arms, heart *(the seat of the emotions)* and ultimately - your brain. By the time you are halfway through the X8 count, visualize **your entire being engulfed by the white light**. At this point you may start to feel dizzy and experience a *head rush*. That is normal; your body may not be accustomed to receiving such a concentrated amount of oxygen. Place all of your mental faculties into this simple visualization. Allow all other distracting thoughts to pass/ use the *Time Trap Escape* to focus on the present moment. Whatever is troubling you at the time ... whether it be negative thoughts, an

emotion or just plain old fashioned hunger – **visualize them being covered and consumed by the white light**.

* When the X8 count is completed, start to **SLOWLY** exhale out of your mouth. **Visualize the exhalation as black air containing everything that is disturbing you.** Take your time and *see* this dark, ugly air being expelled from your body, **taking with it all of the negativity and discomfort**. You are free. Continue to exhale *slowly* and focus on the **black air** coming out of your mouth until the lungs are COMPLETELY empty. The exhalation process should take at least half of the time that it took to inhale. As in the example above, if the X8 inhalation was 56 seconds, then the exhalation should take around 25 seconds. When exhaling, make sure to *blow out* every last bit of air from your lungs, as if you were putting out the candles in a birthday cake. The *black air* visualization should continue up to the very end.

Light and healing in – Darkness and discomfort out. Light and peace in – stress and anger out. Motivation and mental clarity in – hunger pains and

detox symptoms out ... you get the idea.

* Repeat the first three steps until you have given yourself a *break* of at least ten minutes. If you have more time, by all means continue. I usually try to do around five inhalations and exhalations per *DB* session. The longer you do it, the greater the benefit. However, I suggest that, at first, you do no more than three inhalation/exhalations until your body gets used to the exercise. Some people have reported intense lightheadedness when doing this type of intense breathing. So take it easy and work your way up slowly. As you will discover, *DB* is very powerful. I have gone from imminent physical and emotional collapse to restored clarity and motivation with the aid of this simple technique, in combination with the *Time Trap Escape*. At one point I almost broke a 120-day liquid fast out of anger and because I was craving a glazed donut. Ten minutes of *DB* saved the day. Doing it while driving *(with eyes open of course!)* is helpful. Rather than sitting in traffic annoyed, be productive and practice *DB*.

Breathing and Your Health

There are also specific health reasons to practice *DB*. The rhythmic motion of the lungs is very important to expel excess mucus, which can inhibit breathing.

Moreover, **slow deep breathing gets rid of carbon dioxide waste and takes in plenty of clean, fresh oxygen. Blood cells get the new, oxygen-rich air (white light) and the body expels the old stale one (black air).** *DB* helps the body eliminate carbon dioxide much faster than shallow breathing. You'll not only be healthier, but you'll perform better, be less stressed and feel more relaxed. This will help you immensely to handle hunger, cravings and the emotional see-saw incited by the lifestyle changes you are making.

Chapter 14

Choose a Start Date

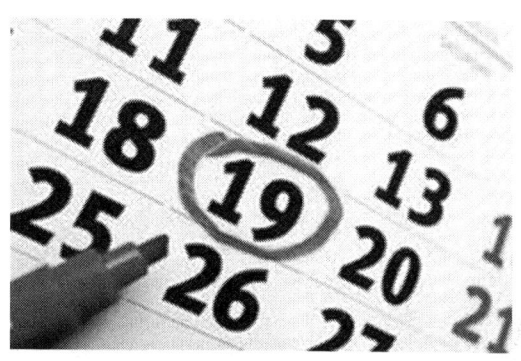

We have set a very thorough foundation. Now it is time for you to choose a date to start the 14-day cleanup and subsequent water fast. This is very exciting. I almost feel as though I am right there with you in person... sharing a moment that - *without a doubt* - is sure to have a great impact on your life.

Right now, we must press on with the task at hand. There is much reward in this, but there is also a lot of challenge. Therefore, the most important step you can take now is to:

Mark your calendar and propose to begin the cleanup no later than 7 days from today.

I like to start on Sundays because it gives

me a straight week-to-week structure. However, your schedule may be different. As a rule, it is preferable to start the cleanup during your *'weekend,'* or whichever time you have weekly of least activity. That way you can get plenty of rest in the initial days before you have to resume any type of work schedule.

<u>IF</u>, you are able to take the <u>entire month</u> off to focus strictly on the cleanup and fasting, by all means do so. If not, then that is fine. I have done plenty of long-term fasts while maintaining an active (*and very demanding*) schedule. It is doable. In some cases, it is even better **because you will be busy and time will go by faster**. So please don't put off this task if you work a full-time job.

If I did it, so can you. You might not have as much energy as you normally would, but you can still make it. Did you choose a start date? Excellent... you have taken yet another step towards the realization of your weight loss and health-improvement goals.

Chapter 15

Intermittent Fasting Alternatives

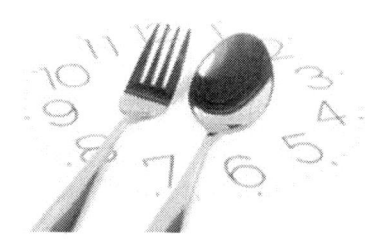

I get into much more detail about intermittent fasting on Volume 2 of this series titled *The Intermittent Fasting Weight Loss Formula*. I encourage you to read that book as well when you have a chance. For guidance, here are some intermittent fasting choices that you can consider. Not everyone may be ready to fast nonstop for an entire 30 days. However, there are shorter fasts that you can practice right away to build experience, strength and confidence. Let's take a look at what these options are:

Daily Intermittent Fasting: As in Catholic Lent Fasting and Muslim Ramadan, here you would fast from sunup to sundown - approximately 12 hours daily. The fast is broken each night with a light meal, preferably of lean fish or poultry, small portion of carbs (*4oz baked or sweet potato, brown rice, multigrain pasta*) and steamed veggies. The *eating window* remains open until dawn, but for most of that time you will be sleeping.

Twelve hours to eat, twelve hours to fast... and so the cycle continues each day. I strongly recommend that you do **NOT** eat anything after *10PM*. Just because you have twelve hours daily to eat doesn't provide license to overeat. You can get up in the *AM*, have a light breakfast (*oatmeal with skim milk, three egg whites and four ounces of ground turkey is my personal favorite*), and then fast for the next 12 hours.

I love Daily (**IF**). It is great for beginners. After acquiring some experience, many like to add hours as they are motivated. In the beginning, you may be adding minutes. That's OK. Minutes add up to hours and hours add up to days.

Remember this motto: *Progress, not perfection*. In other words, certain days you may feel great and want to fast for another few hours. That is fine. But try not to exceed 16 hours of fasting each day, so as to not interrupt the Daily (**IF**) cycle.

Estimated Weekly weight loss: three to five pounds. The key to successful weight loss with *Daily IF* is to eat clean meals; keep the consumption of fat and sugar low. Observe the banned foods!

Every Other Day Intermittent Fasting: Another form of intermittent fasting is to go for an entire 24-hour cycle every other day. Example: You fast from *8AM* Monday morning to *8AM* Tuesday morning. Eat lightly on Tuesday. Wake up on Wednesday at *7:30AM* and have breakfast. Start the fast at 8AM until the same time on Thursday... and so on.

Estimated Weekly weight loss: two to four pounds.

Half Week Intermittent Fasting: Fast for 3.5 days weekly. Example: Fast from *8AM* Monday to 8PM Thursday. You can return to regular eating for the rest of the week. Fasting would resume the following Monday at *8AM* - repeating the same cycle. This system requires caution, however. Since one does not eat for 84-hour periods, it will be necessary to follow the breaking a fast instructions, listed towards the end of this book.

Estimated weekly weight loss: three to five pounds.

Seven Day Intermittent Fasting: Fast for an entire seven days, return to your regular diet for seven days, and then fast for another seven days. Similar to the *Half Week* method, you will need to follow the breaking a fast instructions.

Estimated weekly weight loss: Five to 20 pounds during initial 7-day fast and five to seven on subsequent ones.

Combination Intermittent Fasting: The ultimate way to practice intermittent fasting is to combine all of the above and complete 14 and 30-day intermittent fasts. Whatever is within your ability to do is more than enough to get started. As I said already, what matters is that you jump aboard and get going. A lot of people that have fasted for 14 days and beyond first had to begin with shorter ones to build their confidence. So, if you are experienced and have done it before, then bon voyage - you're on your way. If, on the other hand, you are new to water fasting, then do what you can and build from there. No matter what you are able to do, you come off a winner!

Chapter 16
Water Quality

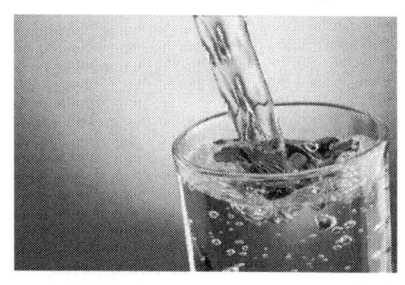

Before we begin the fast, I want to encourage you to get the very best quality of water that you can afford. I definitely discourage the use of tap water, no matter how good the city or county officials say that it is (*I'll tell you why in just a minute*). If, at present, tap water is the best that you can get, then it is imperative that you **boil it for at least ten minutes** before you set it aside for consumption.

Neither do I recommend bottled water because it can get very expensive, not to mention that the disposal of the plastic recipients is terrible for the environment. For those on a tight budget, I would recommend the 4-gallon *Zen Countertop Filter*, a compact, multi-stage filtration system that removes bacteria, harmful contaminants, chlorine, chemicals and other impurities. At $89, you can't beat it; and the water quality is excellent. Another option is the *Aquasana Countertop Filter*; it doesn't have to be installed under the sink and is also quite affordable at $90.

On the other hand, you may opt for a *pitcher purification system* such as the *Brita* or *PUR*, priced at around $30. The problem with pitcher purifiers is that they come in limited sizes, so they have to be constantly refilled. I prefer countertop filters because I can get as much water as I need without waiting for it to travel through the filters.

If, on the other hand, you CAN afford the expense, my top choice would be for you to purchase a *water ionizer*. Ionized water is the purest and most delicious water on planet earth, in my humble opinion. Water ionizers have been used in Japan and other parts of Asia for over 40 years and are certified by the *Korean and Japanese Ministries of Health* as an approved medical device. Ionized water is said to restore the body's pH balance, act as a powerful antioxidant and improve cellular hydration. Furthermore, ionized water is said to help treat a variety of health conditions, including arthritis, digestive system disorders, inflammation, rashes and skin eruptions, obesity, diabetes, cancer, acid reflux, gout, fatigue, allergies, and chronic pain, among others. In short, please use the best quality of water that you can afford.

Your body will be going through an intense process of cleansing and detoxification. You don't want the water that you use to have any pollutants whatsoever but rather be pristine and clear. A bitter situation that I went through some years ago has made me very insistent on using only quality water when fasting (*and otherwise*). In my haste to start fasting, I began to drink from a water fountain at the men's rehab center where I was working as a volunteer. Bad move. It turns out that, during the days that I was there, a parasitic infestation tainted the water sources in the region. Within two days, I was extremely sick with nausea, diarrhea, fever, vomiting and terrible aches and pains. The men's center was located in the mountains, far away from the city. Therefore, it took me nearly three days to get to a hospital and receive medical attention. I was very thin by then, not from fasting and weight loss, but from crapping my brains out non-stop for 48 hours! It was a terrible experience. So I am very leery of any kind of tap or unpurified water. In 2011, the website 247wallst.com inspected water quality in large American cities using data collected by the environmental research and advocacy organization Environmental Working Group from 2004 to 2009. Here are the Top 10 U.S. cities with the worst water quality.

10. Jacksonville, Fla.

Twenty three different toxic chemicals were identified in the water supply. These included *trihalomethanes*, which contains four cleaning byproducts, one of which is chloroform. Many *trihalomethanes* are believed to be carcinogenic. Over the five-year testing period, unsafe levels of *trihalomethanes* were detected during each of the 32 months of testing, and levels deemed illegal by the EPA were detected in 12 of those months. During at least one testing period, *trihalomethane* levels were measured at nearly twice the EPA legal limit. Chemicals like arsenic and lead were also detected at levels exceeding health guidelines.

9. San Diego (San Diego Water Department)

According to California's Department of Public Health, San Diego's drinking water system contained eight chemicals exceeding health guidelines as well as two chemicals that exceeded the EPA's legal limit. In total, 20 contaminants have been found. One of those in excess of the EPA limit was *trihalomethanes*. The other was manganese, a natural element that's a byproduct of industrial manufacturing and can be poisonous to humans.

8. North Las Vegas (City of North Las Vegas Utilities Department)

North Las Vegas's water supply mostly comes from groundwater and the Colorado River, and doesn't contain chemicals exceeding legal limits. However, the water supply did contain 11 chemicals that exceeded health guidelines set by federal and state health agencies. The national average for chemicals found in cities' water exceeding health guidelines is four. North

Las Vegas had a total of 26 contaminants, compared with the national average of eight. The water contained an extremely high level of uranium, a radioactive element.

7. Omaha (Metropolitan Utilities District)

The land-locked city of Omaha gets its water from the Missouri and Platte Rivers, as well as from groundwater. Of the 148 chemicals tested for in Omaha, 42 were detected in some amount, 20 of which were above health guidelines, and four of those were detected in illegal amounts. These were atrazine, *trihalomethanes*, nitrate and nitrite, and manganese. Atrazine is an herbicide that has been shown to cause birth defects. Nitrate is found in fertilizer, and nitrite is used for curing meat. Manganese was detected at 40 times the legal limit during one month of testing.

6. Houston (City of Houston Public Works)

Houston is the fourth-largest U.S. city. It gets its water from sources such as the Trinity River, the San Jacinto Rivers and

Lake Houston. Texas conducted 22,083 water quality tests between 2004 and 2007 on Houston's water supply, and found 18 chemicals that exceeded federal and state health guidelines, compared to the national average of four. Three chemicals exceeded EPA legal health standards, against the national average of 0.5 chemicals. A total of 46 pollutants were detected, compared to the national average of eight. The city water has contained illegal levels of alpha particles, a form of radiation. Similarly, *haloacetic acids*, from various disinfection byproducts, have been detected.

5. Reno (Truckee Meadows Water Authority)

Reno gets most of its water from the Truckee River, which flows from Lake Tahoe. Of the 126 chemicals tested for in Reno over four years, 21 were discovered in the city's water supply, eight of which were detected in levels above EPA health guidelines, and three of these occurred in illegal amounts. These were *manganese, tetrachloroethylene and arsenic. Tetrachloroethylene* is a fluid used for dry cleaning and as an industrial solvent, and is deemed a likely carcinogenic by the International Agency for Research on Cancer. Arsenic is a byproduct of herbicides and pesticides, and is extremely poisonous to humans. During at least one month of testing, arsenic levels were detected at roughly two and a half times the legal limit.

4. Riverside County, Calif. (Eastern Municipal Water District)

Riverside county is a 7,200-square-mile area located north of San Diego, part of California's "Inland Empire." The county is primarily located in desert territory, and so the water utilities draw their supply from the Bay Delta, which is miles to the north. The water in Riverside County contained 13 chemicals that exceeded recommended health guidelines over the four tested years, and one that exceeded legal limits. In total, 22 chemicals were detected in the district's water supply. The contaminant exceeding legal health standards was *tetrachloroethylene.*

3. Las Vegas (Las Vegas Valley Water District)

Located in the Mojave Desert, Las Vegas

gets its water from the Colorado River through miles-long intake pipes. While its water doesn't exceed the legal limits for any single type of contaminant, Las Vegas's water has a large range of pollutants. Of the 125 chemicals tested for over a five-year period, 30 were identified in some amount, and 12 were found in levels that exceeded EPA health guidelines. These chemicals included radium-226, radium-228, arsenic and lead. The two radium isotopes are commonly found around uranium deposits and are hazardous to human health, even in small quantities.

2. Riverside, Calif. (City of Riverside Public Utilities)

Riverside, with a population slightly greater than 300,000, gets most of its drinking supply from groundwater. Regulators in the city of Riverside, which has a different water-treatment facility than the rest of Riverside County, detected 15 chemicals that exceeded health guidelines and one that exceeded legal standards. In total, 30 chemicals were found. Since 2004, the water has almost consistently been riddled with alpha particle activity, traces of bromoform (a form of trihalomethane) and uranium, causing an unusually unhealthy water supply.

1. Pensacola, Fla. (Emerald Coast Water Utility)

Located on the Florida Panhandle along the Gulf of Mexico, Pensacola is Florida's westernmost major city. Analysts say it has the worst water quality in the country. Of the 101 chemicals tested for over five years, 45 were discovered. Of them, 21 were discovered in unhealthy amounts. The worst of these were radium-228 and -228, trichloroethylene, tetrachloroethylene, alpha particles, benzine and lead. Pensacola's water was also found to contain cyanide and chloroform. The combination of these chemicals makes Pensacola's water supply America's most unhealthy.

Source: dailyfinance.com January 31, 2011.

I certainly do not give you this information to scare you. I do, however, want you to be aware that tap water can have contaminants. Is the quality of tap water good in your city? Probably yes. Maybe no. Do you know for sure? Please do not assume that the water is fine. Rather, err in the side of caution; purchase the best water filtration that you can afford. As I said, the body goes through an intense process of detoxification while fasting. Why throw a wrench into it by drinking substandard water?

Bottom line:

If you don't already have a reliable and effective water filtration system, then take your time and purchase one before you start this fast.

Chapter 17

Starting the Fast

From this point onward I will assume that you completed the 14-day preparation phase and are ready to begin water fasting - tomorrow. So today is the last day of your *'pre-fasting'* life. You are moving towards what I call *'The Land of Miracles.'* The possibilities for your life are vast. You've worked hard and made it this far. Now we're about to dive into the deep, healing waters.

Are you with me? Spend some time today writing in your journal. Get used to recording your thoughts and feelings; **your journal is one of the most powerful weapons that you have**. Use it constantly; it will feed you with strength and inspiration when you need it the most. Now let's gaze directly at the task at hand – **30 days of water fasting**. You may have been insecure or intimidated in the past, but today you look at your journey with hope and optimism. You feel a rush of righteous anger pulsating through your veins. This is constructive anger! Why? Because it gives you unusual strength and determination to do **whatever it takes** to reach your objective.

The mind gives you a brief tour of your failures; how you tried to lose weight many times yet fell short, how your eating patterns have become more and more disorganized, how you dream of reaching your ideal weight but, up to now, have lacked the discipline and commitment to make it happen. And so, righteous anger surges from the deepest parts of your soul; it travels up your stomach, to your vocal chords where, in a cathartic moment, it cries out: "NEVER AGAIN! NEVER AGAIN! NEVER AGAIN!"

That is the cry of the fasting warrior; **hearts groaning in unison, pledging to overcome weaknesses, resolving to go all the way!** Your heart now burns with courage, self-assurance and steadfastness; NOTHING can stop you from reaching your goal. This is your moment of transcendence, your time of triumph! *Hunger pangs and detox symptoms, the once large and looming foes that threatened to knock you off the race, are now but tiny mice without teeth. They no longer have any power over you; they never did.* Therefore, I entreat you, walk through the 30 days of water fasting with your head held high, and take each step with the certainty that, this time, you **WILL** reach your ideal weight. And there's good reason to be optimistic: You have powerful artillery at your disposal. You did the 14-day preparation period, so your body has already begun to burn fat and detoxify.

In addition, you were introduced to some simple but effective mental tricks and techniques that will help you to confront and vanquish hunger and detox symptoms. Remember what they were? **The Anchor Questions** (*the answers should be constantly expanded*), **The Time-Trap Escape** (*which use the senses of sight and sound to forcefully draw your attention to the immediate present*), **The Five D's** (*decide, define, declare, designate and develop*) and, my personal favorite, **Detox**

Breathing (*an intensive breathing/visualization exercise designed to expel toxins from the body and help refresh a tired or troubled mind*). When used appropriately, these weapons will ALWAYS help you beat hunger and detox symptoms (*as well as any other emotional uprisings that surface during the fast*). But you have received more: You've learned how **Green Tea** can give you a pep of energy in the afternoons, how **Seltzer Wat**er (*sparkling water/club soda*) helps to soothe hunger and reduce the intensity of many detox symptoms, and how fasting-induced insomnia can be counteracted with a *500mg* tablet of **Tryptophan** or two **Valerian Root** capsules. With all of these tools within your grasp, how could you possibly fail?

The only way that you will fail is if you become mentally distracted and allow the mind to deceive you into breaking the fast prematurely. There are, of course, legitimate reasons for halting the program as, for example, strong detox symptoms that do not go away after several days, the emergence of unexplained symptoms (*pain, bleeding, inflammation*), having to travel overseas to handle a delicate business situation, the discovery that *Halley's Comet* is on a direct trajectory with planet Earth and/or hundreds of *UFOs* appearing in the clouds all over the world. What I mean is this: If it isn't a direct emergency related to your health or your loved ones, there really is **ZERO** reason for you to break this fast once you start!

And so I now invite you to recite the *'warrior's mindset.'* Repeat out loud:

"This day, I make an unshakable commitment with myself to go all the way and do whatever it takes to accomplish my goals! I will hang on for 30 days! I will hang on for 30 days! No matter what! No matter what! No matter what! I will not stop! I will hang on for 30 days! No matter what! No matter what! No matter what! I will not stop! Rain or shine, hunger or detox symptoms, I will hang on for 30 days! No matter what! No matter what! I will not stop!"

Repeat the *warrior's mindset* several times per day. Use it whenever you feel tired, emotional and/or vulnerable. The more you can tap into that message of triumph and optimism, the easier it will be to deal with hunger and physical discomfort. Don't allow negativity to enter into your mind; it will always try to sneak in to influence your mood and emotions. Don't let it! Read the *warrior's mindset* and let those words fill your heart and mind with courage, strength, hope and inevitable triumph. Any thought or emotion that tries to weaken you or bring pain and/or confusion, get rid of it. How? By going back to and reciting the *warrior's mindset*. I think you get the idea. Spend as much time as possible practicing the **Time-Trap Escape** and **Detox Breathing**.

At first some of it may not make sense, especially this concept about being *'trapped in time.'* But the more you practice it, the faster it will *'click'* in your mind and open you to a whole new level of awareness. Here's my message for you: *The amazing gift of weight loss, health and life is at your fingertips, and nothing will keep you from seizing it ever again. You are ready!* Let's move forward with the motivational messages, starting on **Day 0** which is <u>**TODAY**</u>, the day before the fast.

Chapter 18

Motivational Messages

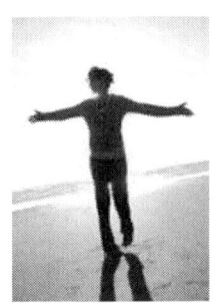

The motivational messages in this section will guide you through the first 10 days of fasting. Read each one in the morning and keep referring to them throughout the day. If anything in the messages strikes you as significant, take out your journal and write about it.

Once you reach day 10, return to the first message and go through the sequence all over again. There actually are a total of 11 messages, starting with *Day 0*, the day BEFORE you start the fast.

In addition to the motivational messages, you also have a wealth of material available to you via the *Fasting Masterclass*. If you haven't already done so, visit the **Sign in Page** (http://www.fitnessthroughfasting.com/post-purchase-thanks.html) and download all six modules. You'll also see various mind maps and .PDF bonus reports; if anything catches your eye, by all means grab it. There's a lot of material in that download page; I suggest that you spend some time there **NOW** and become familiar with the content. That way, once you start fasting, you'll know which topics are discussed in which modules.

I don't know about you, but I'm a total computer slob. My desktop is crammed with icons and files of every sort, many of which I haven't used in years. Consequently, when there's a file that I really need, it often takes me a bit of time to locate it. When fasting, that type of delay can easily result in a relapse. Therefore, I suggest that you create a new folder (*in your desktop or documents directory*) and name it *'fasting* **masterclass**.'

As you download the material from the member's area, simply save it to this new folder; nice and easy. You want to have quick access to any and all of this material; you never know when something that I say is going to give you that push that you needed to keep going. So keep the **masterclass** material organized and handy. The motivational messages that I've written are great, but loading those *mp3s* and having my voice in your ear will be much more helpful. Start with *Module 1* and just keep going from there; listen (*or view*) the modules over and over. *Listen to my voice until you get sick of it!* Then keep listening, day and night if necessary. One lady wrote me a few months ago to tell me that she had never been able to fast for longer than three days. This time, however, she loaded the masterclass *mp3s* on her *iPhone* and listened to the material all day long. When hunger pangs and detox symptoms came around to bother her, she said she would put on her ear buds and listen to my presentation. In this fashion, she said she was able to complete ten full days of fasting, something she had tried many times but had never accomplished. So, by all means, use the *masterclass* material to keep your mind busy and engaged in the topic. Furthermore, don't forget to visit the Fasting Forum, sign up for your free account and begin to post regularly. You will find much support and encouragement from others who are also in the fasting path.

Day 0 - Day Before Starting the Fast

The fact that you are reading these words shows that you are committed to doing whatever it takes to improving your health and quality of life. Am I right? Did you complete the 14-day Pre-Fasting Phase? If you did, then I congratulate you and give you major kudos! How did it go? How did you make out with the menu and the meals?

Getting good at creating menus and preparing meals has been key in keeping me thin and binge-free for more than 10 years.

So even if you *'hate cooking,'* get over it and do it anyways! It gets easier with time, and you will feel very gratified with the results. I am very proud of you. Completing those 14 days of preparation is a huge accomplishment. Now it is time to press forward and begin the 30-day water fast. How are you feeling? Do you feel calm and confident, or a little nervous? If you are a tad nervous, that's fine... I myself was **VERY** nervous before I started my first long-term water fast. But we are the kind of people who take action in spite of nervousness, right? In addition, what is really scary is to

DO NOTHING and never reach our goals. That is definitely something to be nervous about. But, no more! That is not going to happen, right? I ask you: Are you prepared to put to practice everything that we have learned? Are you ready to see this **all the way through**? I believe that you are! If you have never fasted before, you are in for quite the ride.

If you <u>HAVE</u> done long-term fasts, then I am certain you will learn even more; *every fast is unique and has its own set of lessons to teach.* So this is the moment of truth. **Tomorrow you begin your fast.** You have everything that you need to cross the finish line; you have a lot more than I did when I first started fasting. Believe me, back then, I would have been immensely happy to have these tools that I've shared with you. All I had was my sheer determination to overcome obesity and binging. A lot of those initial times of fasting were very lonely and difficult. Apart from my mentor *John Benitez*, I was alone. But I can see now how those dark moments were necessary. It was in those rough spots (*stricken with intense hunger and detox symptoms*) that I learned most of the material that I now share with you. By directly confronting hunger and detox symptoms, I got to know myself at a much deeper level. When I let go of my fear of discomfort, I found myself not only learning to handle hunger and detox symptoms, but actually being able to disconnect them completely. How? By relentlessly practicing the **Time Trap Escape** and **Detox Breathing**. I also spend a lot of time meditating when I'm fasting. If you do the *Time Trap Escape and Detox Breathing* together, you will find a really deep and cozy place in which to meditate. Give it a shot; practice it and you'll see what I mean.

Cleaning House

Ok, now it is time to do a house cleanup. No, I don't mean dusting or mopping, although I do often get into *'cleaning mode'* while fasting to kill time and keep myself occupied. The cleanup that I'm referring to here is **emptying the house of any and all junk foods and beverages that may be left in the cupboards, drawers and/or refrigerator, among other places.** Ask your loved ones to please *'hide'* their treats and other such foods, that you are trying to lose weight and need their help. In most cases, family members are happy to oblige; they will be delighted to know that you are taking action to improve your health. But you must make sure that the house is as clean and free of tempting food as possible. Go through the entire kitchen and remove the offending foods; *out of sight, out of mind.*

This is very important. Do not skip this step. One gentleman that I worked with some years ago was doing great; he had reached day 21 of water fasting and had lost more than 30 pounds. But he did not do the house cleanup as I suggested. One afternoon, while he was navigating a tough wave of hunger, he opened the cupboard and found two boxes of corn and bran muffins, smiling and fervently calling his name. *"Charles! Charles! Come to us Charles!"*

He was vulnerable and, in spite of the amazing progress he had made, he opened the boxes and ate all 9 muffins. He called me in tears, feeling defeated and demoralized, not to mention that he fell ill;

breaking a long fast inappropriately is very dangerous and could result in serious injury and even death. He had to go to the hospital and have his stomach pumped because the digestive system had been hibernating and could not handle the sudden intake of food. That incident could have been avoided if only Charles had been willing to follow some simple instructions. And I confess that the same thing happened to me when I first started fasting. I was on day 14 of a water fast and went to visit a friend. As soon as I walked in I saw the dining room table full of pizzas of different flavors. The smell was intoxicating. Rather than turn around and leave (*the appropriate course of action*), I toyed with the idea and eventually gave in. I ate like five slices (*more like inhaled them*). Within half an hour, my face and belly began to swell and I started to vomit violently.

When I looked at myself in the mirror I saw dark (*nearly black*) circles around my eyes. My friends had to call 911. And there I was, in front of all of those pretty girls, being strapped to a stretcher and hauled away like the idiot that I was. Turns out that eating the pizza nearly ruptured the linings of my stomach; I would have died. So don't skip the cleanup please; take the time, go through your home and remove all trigger foods (*or have your loved ones hide it*). That is a smart military offensive; when you're in double digits of fasting, the last thing you want is to battle with a muffin that was left carelessly on the kitchen table. Of course, that isn't to say that everyone has to treat you with *'kid gloves'* because you're so weak and ready to fall to pieces. No. Life is life, and there may be times when you'll have to face plates of delicious food while fasting. That is when you have to go back to your journal and reinforce in your mind the reasons why you are doing this.

That reminds me of one of the first times that I did a 30-day water fast. I was in the mountains in Puerto Rico at a men's rehab center working as a volunteer. I drove up there, got out of my truck and walked to the office where I met Angel, the director. "Oh, here's our new cook," he said with a mischievous smile. I thought I was going to have a coronary. "What!" I replied, agitated. "What do you mean cook? You know that I came here to fast!" It was no use; turns out, the guy who was supposed to be the cook got sick and was unable to come. I was stuck with the job. What was the job? To prepare three meals a day for 50 men, and to do it all while water fasting. To say that it was a major test is an understatement. But I made it. How? Lots of *Time Trap Escape*, lots of *Detox Breathing*, lots of *journaling*, lots of *green tea*, lots of *seltzer water* and lots of *prayer*. My point is this:

A plate of delicious food or a muffin should not be enough to cause you to collapse, **IF** you have **sufficiently-strong reasons** in your journal. Nevertheless, making sure that the home is free and clear of junk food and any other trigger foods is still a wise step. Make sure to do it at some point today. Alright! **For today**: Have your last meal at around 8PM, drink two large glasses of water and go to bed. We will make it... just one moment, one day at a time. Get plenty of rest tonight. I will talk to you in the morning!

Day 1

We are off and running. The first day is one of adapting physically and mentally. You ate your final meal last night, so you already have been fasting for at least 12 hours. That means that hunger will come very soon. Be ready! Before we go any further, please stop reading and go drink two large glasses of water. Make it a point to drink at least half a gallon daily, one gallon would be even better! **Water is your ally** and will help soothe hunger and detox symptoms.

How are you feeling? Where is your mind today? Spend some time and write in your journal, do your customary prayers. Let's recite the *warrior's mindset*. Repeat out loud:

"This day, I make an unshakable commitment with myself to go all the way and do whatever it takes to accomplish my goals! I will hang on for 30 days! I will hang on for 30 days! No matter what! No matter what! No matter what! I will not stop! I will hang on for 30 days! No matter what! No matter what! No matter what! I will not stop! Rain or shine, hunger or detox symptoms, I will hang on for 30 days! No matter what! No

matter what! I will not stop!"

Go through the answers to the *'anchor questions.'* Those are important because, there, you have recorded the specific reasons why completing this fast is important to **YOU**. We need to keep those reasons front and center in our minds at all times. Never go anywhere without your journal and the **masterclass** *mp3's*. If you have to go out to work, I suggest that you take with you a small cooler with ice, several bottles filled with water, three or four green tea envelopes and a few bottles of seltzer water (*sparkling water/club soda*). You need to understand that your daily life is going to be a bit different while you are fasting. If carrying a cooler around bothers you, get over it and do it anyways.

Seriously, **the number one priority right now is your water, tea and seltzer.** I want you to drink from only *one source* of water if at all possible. If you have a good water filtration system at home, then fill plastic bottles and refrigerate them. Remember what happened to me because I trusted the tap water in that rehabilitation center. I'm not saying that the same is going to happen to you. The odds are in your favor that it won't happen. But please be careful. Stick to one source of water, is my recommendation. By around noon, hunger will begin to peek its ugly head. Drink two large glasses of water; crack open a bottle of seltzer. At around *1:00* or *2:00PM*, have a cup of green tea; it will give you an energy boost as well as calm hunger and symptoms. Try to stay busy, but take it easy physically. Brace yourself; as the afternoon continues, the hunger pangs will get stronger.

Drink more water, seltzer and green tea, but never exceed four seltzer waters daily or three cups of green tea. Green tea has some caffeine, so you don't want to drink it too late in the afternoon or it may keep you up at night. In the afternoon (*around 16-18 hours after you last ate*), you also may start to feel detox symptoms; weakness, dizziness, nausea, headaches, irritability, white coat on the tongue and/or a metallic taste in your mouth. Drink more water, seltzer... green tea. **Move slowly, take a nap if you can**. On average, hunger and symptoms will diminish (*and even vanish*) after roughly *7 to 9* days of water fasting. If you find yourself feeling weak, immediately go to your journal. Remind yourself why you are fasting, and why you are choosing to complete this process. This is **NOT** a game or some half-measured step. You have specific (*and strong*) reasons for doing this, and it has to do with transforming **your life for the better**, right? You want to lose weight, get healthy and rejuvenate! Make sure to speak to your **DECLARE** and **DESIGNATE** support buddy at some point during the day. I have found that afternoons are best because that is the time when hunger and symptoms hit me the most. This entire fast will go by faster and smoother is you have someone who supports and is there for you (*apart from me!*).

Please follow this suggestion. You won't regret it. All in all, after two weeks you should be feeling a lot better. So keep that target in mind as you move forward. Stick to the plan; I'll be here with you. Don't just read this message **ONCE** and then move on. Use it! Read it, read it, read it! There is no more time to waste. This is **YOUR** time. This is the time of your change and transformation. And it has already begun.

Remember, that "*discomfort is a sign that you are getting better*". It doesn't feel good, but the health and weight loss benefits that will result make this "*small sacrifice*" worth its weight in gold! In the evening, watch TV, read a book, write some closing thoughts on your journal.

Drink a cup of chamomile tea to help you relax and get ready for bed. During the initial days of fasting, it is common to go through some bouts of insomnia. The reason for that is that the process of ketosis causes large amounts of toxins to be released into the bloodstream. The healing crisis we talked about earlier ensues, and that sometimes makes it hard to fall (*and stay*) asleep. If you find yourself in that situation, take one *500mg Tryptophan*. That works like a charm with me. Within 30 minutes of taking it, I'm out cold. But only use *Tryptophan* if you really need it. If you find that you can sleep just fine on your own, then that is optimal. No reason to take any pills if you don't need them. Remember that you also have chamomile tea and Valerian Root to calm you and help you rest. Do **NOT** take more than two Tryptophan tablets or more than three Valerian Root tablets daily. When I have severe insomnia, I take two Tryptophan and two Valerian Root tablets; in less than 20 minutes I'm cutting serious logs. But please do not take more than that in any given night. If worse comes to worse and you still cannot sleep, then I suggest that you get up and go for a walk (*if it is safe*). **OR**, you can read for a while, **OR** listen to the *masterclass* content. Insomnia doesn't last very long, so do not be discouraged. You're doing great!

Right now, say to yourself: *"Just for today, no matter what, no matter what, no matter what, I am **NOT** going to eat. I am going to stick to my fast and I am going to finish what I started. I thank the God of my understanding for giving me the strength and resolve I need to make it. I am grateful that fasting will make me healthier, leaner and more vibrant so I can be more effective and useful to my loved ones and others."*

Day 2

Welcome to **DAY TWO** of your 30-day fast. I hope you got plenty of sleep. I find that, when I fast, I sleep very deeply and wake up refreshed. Some people, however, go through periods of insomnia, restlessness and even nightmares. As I said, this is due to the **release of toxins into the bloodstream; it will pass**.

As you did yesterday, drink two large glasses of water as soon as you wake up. Drinking plenty of water during the day will help to expedite the *flushing out* of toxins from your body. In most cases, hunger is minimal when you first wake up. Enjoy it. Over the following hours, however, you will notice the pangs increasing, so **be very careful**. Remain vigilant. It is during this early phase that many tend to give up. As usual, sit on the kitchen table, write on your journal and do your customary prayers (if any). How are you feeling today? Where is your mind? Let's dive right in and do the *warrior's mindset*. Repeat out loud:

"This day, I make an unshakable commitment with myself to go all the way and do whatever it takes to accomplish my

goals! I will hang on for 30 days! I will hang on for 30 days! No matter what! No matter what! No matter what! I will not stop! I will hang on for 30 days! No matter what! No matter what! No matter what! I will not stop! Rain or shine, hunger or detox symptoms, I will hang on for 30 days! No matter what! No matter what! I will not stop!"

Many times the words will be powerful and they will give you a jolt of encouragement and motivation. Other times, they may seem totally silly and ineffective. That's fine; keep doing it anyways. We want to keep driving the message home to the subconscious mind that we are not playing games with this, but that we are prepared to go all the way. Today, apart from the physical symptoms, pay close attention to your mind and emotions. Learn to identify and reject all thoughts, arguments, rationalizations and justifications the mind may give you to give up.

Resistance, resistance, resistance is key at this phase! None of the discomfort should come as a big shock. We knew it would be a challenge; you can make it through. I know that you can. **DAY TWO** is nearly-always a day of battle. But you know what you have to do. Write in your journal, listen to the masterclass *mp3's*, practice the **Time Trap Escape** and **Detox Breathing**, continue to expand your answers to the *'anchor questions.'* Keep your mind busy and drink water constantly. Write, read, pray, meditate... whatever it takes to keep you moving forward. Visit the **Fasting Forum** and find as many people as you can to motivate and comfort. It never ceases to amaze me just how powerful this simple practice is.

You can be struggling with hunger and/or detox symptoms, yet a few minutes of writing to help someone else will strengthen and refresh you. The more time you spend *'giving'* strength, the more you will receive!

Not to mention that you will find plenty of people there to support and comfort you as well. Those forums are immensely helpful. Go there daily and get involved. You may even find me there! Every time, every moment that hunger and detox symptoms disturb you, remember this:

YOU ARE NOT GOING THROUGH THE DISCOMFORT IN VAIN!

<u>You have a plan and you have the courage</u>. You are taking control of your life and squashing <u>anything</u> that stands in your way.

You are adding quality years to your life and bravely going through the road less traveled.

Every symptom <u>**MUST**</u> yield to your resolve. This, without a doubt, is one of the most important moments in your life. Do you see it! Can you internalize the <u>**HUGE**</u> magnitude of what you are doing? Try to take it easy if you are able. Stay busy but <u>do not</u> put yourself through unnecessary exertion. You may start to experience some mood *swings now; irritability, sadness, hopelessness, anger, rage... these are all symptoms that you are getting better.*

The toxins are being wiped out and your mind and emotions are undergoing a process of purging and healing. Thank the God of your understanding and ask for strength to make it through. This is <u>**NOT**</u> just about losing weight and external physical health. You also have put yourself in a position to undergo profound emotional healing and spiritual growth. The benefits are huge! **The symptoms will**

pass. The hurricane will weaken. You will reach the shore a stronger and more vibrant person.

Say to yourself: *"Just for today, I will keep in mind that I am undergoing a physical, mental and spiritual cleansing and will not react when I feel bad. I will let the symptoms and feelings pass and keep my eyes <u>ONLY</u> on reaching my goals. I will ask the God of my understanding for help and be empowered by my choice to live a better life."*

Day 3

DAY THREE! Seventy-two hours... you are entering deeper and deeper waters. How have you been feeling? Have you been drinking plenty of water? Have you been writing in your journal? Did you call your **DESIGNATE** friend? If you have, then good for you! That shows commitment, courage and willingness. You will be greatly rewarded mentally, physically and, yes, spiritually.

Nothing kills our progress more than procrastination and closed-mindedness. So give yourself completely to this fast. I cannot overestimate the power that it will unleash in your life. Today can either be the toughest day of the fast, or it can be the day when one begins to feel better. It all depends on how your body reacts. But you are gaining ground. The digestive system is slowing down considerably and the body is starting to feed more and more on stored fat.

Ketosis is almost complete (*the process where the body shifts from feeding on food intake, to feeding mostly on stored fat*). Drink your customary two large glasses of water upon awakening, and sit down to write on your journal; do your customary devotional and, by all means, start listening to the *masterclass* material. There are various '*homework*' reports on the *masterclass*; download them and start to work on those as well. Visit the **Fasting Forum** and write a post about how you are feeling and the progress you are making. Later in the afternoon, you can go back and check for responses and write another post. The more connected you remain to a fasting community, the easier this entire process will be. Meanwhile, make sure that you have enough seltzer and green tea to carry you through the day. Those are your allies and we do not want to run short.

How did you sleep? In the first days of fasting, it is not unusual to wake up several times during the night. Sometimes the hunger can be quite strong. Stay away from the kitchen. **NEVER** enter the kitchen for any reason. Keep a supply of water in your bedroom and drink from it. Entering the kitchen and opening the refrigerator is a bad idea at this point. If you live with others, there's no telling what type of foods you may see that could trigger a response. If you find yourself awake in the middle of the night, drink two large glasses of water; take two *Valerian Root* capsules and listen to the *masterclass* material until you fall back asleep. Overall, how are you feeling this morning? Let's waste no time. The *warrior's mindset* shows us the way. Repeat out loud:

"This day, I make an unshakable commitment with myself to go all the way and do whatever it takes to accomplish my goals! I will hang on for 30 days! I will hang on for 30 days! No matter what! No matter what! No matter what! I will not stop! I will hang on for 30 days! No matter what! No matter what! No matter what! I will not stop! Rain or shine, hunger or detox symptoms, I will hang on for 30 days! No matter what! No matter what! I will not stop!"

Stay away from food and eating establishments as much as possible.

This is a crucial time in the fast. The worst of the toxins are being eliminated; that is what causes the symptoms and the hunger pangs. You **KNOW** why you are doing this. You are determined to make it to the other side. You are tired of talking about it and wishing and sighing... *"You are prepared to take the action and to stay the course until you produce the results that you want"*. Am I right? Your body is busy cleansing and healing.

All you have to do is stay put and give it the time it needs to complete the process.

The weight loss accelerates today. The body is shifting to *"full fat-burning mode"* and a lot of toxins are being eliminated, along with the normal water weight loss. The toxins that have been hiding in stored fat are being exposed and wiped out. You, your body *and the God of your understanding* are working together to vanquish these enemies and achieve ultimate health and breakthrough. And I am here cheering you on; filling **your mind with powerful thoughts and motivation!**

Say to yourself: *"Just for today, I am going to surrender to the process and give my body the time that it needs to heal and cleanse. I thank the God of my understanding that I have been given the knowledge and strength I need to make it through these 24 hours. I am at peace and in full expectation of greater* *and greater blessings."*

Day 4

Hello dear friend, and welcome to day 4! It is very possible that today the hunger and detox symptoms will begin to subside. **OR**, as is the case with me, you may be in the middle of the storm and struggling to hang on. But you have the willingness to work through this challenge. I encourage you to spend as much time as possible in your journal and listening to the *masterclass* content. We are not out of the woods yet and need to use everything at our disposal to make it from day to day.

Good news: **Your body will reach full *Ketosis* today**. For many people, the hunger and detox symptoms are starting to subside. How are you feeling? Waking up with little or no hunger is one of the most rewarding times. Have you experienced that? If you have <u>NOT</u> felt any improvement and are struggling, just hang on! **It will pass, it will pass, and it will pass! Did I mention also that it will pass?**

Let's continue to reinforce the *warrior's mindset!* Repeat out loud:

"This day, I make an unshakable

commitment with myself to go all the way and do whatever it takes to accomplish my goals! I will hang on for 30 days! I will hang on for 30 days! No matter what! No matter what! No matter what! I will not stop! I will hang on for 30 days! No matter what! No matter what! No matter what! I will not stop! Rain or shine, hunger or detox symptoms, I will hang on for 30 days! No matter what! No matter what! I will not stop!"

Just hang on, put on your armor and continue offering full **RESISTANCE**. Enough is enough right? You're **NOT** going to let the years keep going by without achieving your ideal weight and health, right? Get tough... get angry! What is going through your mind today? Are you spending time in your fasting journal? You are now in the midst of the full power of fasting. You are going deeper and deeper into the land of miracles. Your spirit is more awake than ever ... whatever your spiritual belief, **NOW** is an amazingly-powerful moment to have communion with the *God of your understanding.* Spending more time in your accustomed prayers and/or meditation is highly encouraged. Optimize water intake today. Make it a point to drink a **FULL** gallon of water daily for the remainder of the fast. You may already be drinking that much. If so, then keep doing it. If not, then today I want you to push yourself and force some more water down. Let's increase the flushing power flowing through your organs. Let's continue to support the body's fat-burning mission. Wherever you go, don't forget to carry your cooler with water and seltzer. **Don't forget to take plenty of green tea to help you with energy.**

Be careful when getting up and moving. The weakness at this point of the fast may be very noticeable. You will probably feel **dizzy and may have difficulty getting around.** Rest is the best alternative. If you must move, do so slowly and do **NOT** make any sudden jerky movements. **Mental confusion and fogginess is also normal.** The cleansing is deep and dramatic ... do not become discouraged.

We already talked about detox symptoms, but let me list them here again for your immediate reference.

Headaches
Dizziness

Difficulty Performing Basic Tasks
Weakness
Pulsating Hunger Pains
Bad Breath
Metallic Taste in Mouth
White Sticky Film on the Tongue
Diarrhea or Constipation
Diarrhea
Constipation
Irritability / Mood Swings

Facial Puffiness & Feeling Bloated

I know that this list looks quite intimidating. The good news is that most of the symptoms listed here barely last more than a few hours or days. You may not experience many of them at all. It all depends on how toxic your body is and the overall condition of your digestive system. What you have to keep in mind is that detox symptoms are good. They may not feel great, but they are a sign that your body is getting cleaner and healthier. Help the body by drinking lots and lots of water. In those initial days of detoxification, I sometimes use a light herbal laxative called *Herbs & Prunes* to completely empty the digestive system and incite maximum cleansing. That is my personal choice and it works great because it doubles and triples the intensity of each bowel movement. After a few of those, I'm barking at the moon for sure! At any rate, if you wish to try Herbs & Prunes, use only one tablet and see what happens. Never take more than four at a time. .

Say to yourself: *"Just for today, I am going to stay on my fast no matter what my mind and body tell me. Today I am going to keep in mind constantly just how important this is to me and how many wonderful benefits I am gaining by staying the path. I thank the God of my understanding for giving me the strength and courage that I need. I trust the amazing task my body is doing on my behalf"*.

Day 5

WOW, DAY FIVE! You are amazing. How is it going? Each passing moment brings you closer to your ultimate goal. Did you speak to your **DESIGNATE** buddy and visit any forums? This is a priority. If you haven't done it, then please make sure to do so starting today. None of us are supermen. We need each other, and that is what the forums are all about. **Please follow my instructions**. Remember that <u>I have gone through this road before</u>. S

o whatever I ask you to do, it isn't *'just because.'* I am asking you to do it because I have walked the path and know that it works. As usual, drink two large glasses of water when you wake up, then sit down to write on your journal and do your usual devotionals. Listen to the *masterclass* content and don't forget to visit the *Fasting Forum*. Post at least two messages daily in the forum. You will find people there who will support you and encourage you in more ways than what you can imagine.

Ok, let's strengthen our mental focus and vision with the *warrior's mindset!* Repeat out loud:

"This day, I make an unshakable commitment with myself to go all the way and do whatever it takes to accomplish my goals! I will hang on for 30 days! I will hang on for 30 days! No matter what! No matter what! No matter what! I will not stop! I will hang on for 30 days! No matter what! No matter what! No matter what! I will not stop! Rain or shine, hunger or detox symptoms, I will hang on for 30 days! No matter what! No matter what! I will not stop!"

Did you drink an entire gallon of water yesterday as I asked you? Make sure to do that, even if you do not feel thirsty or your body does not want it. Water intake is a crucial part of the cleansing process and it also helps expedite the passing of the detox symptoms. Day **FIVE** can often be a day of much weakness, dizziness and medium-to-strong hunger pains. Although, in many cases hunger and symptoms have diminished by now. How is it going with you? What would you say is causing the most discomfort; detox? Hunger? Both? Make sure to write all of this information down in your fasting journal. That will give you excellent insight of how your body reacts when fasting. When you do another long-term fast in the future, you will know what to expect. Such information is invaluable. So write, write, write! Today I want you to spend as much time as possible writing in the journal and listening to the <u>masterclass</u>.

Just put pen to paper and start to write what is in your heart and mind. You are amidst a dynamic program of change. NOW is an amazing time. We are reflecting on the past, present and future. What you are going through is but **a tiny micro in comparison to the large scheme of things and your life as a whole**. In fact, the discomfort that you may be feeling has the potential to "*make the remaining years of your life drastically-more vibrant and effective*". Keep your eyes on **THAT** prize. It is more than a prize... **it is a treasure**! Again, you are **NOT** walking through the discomfort of fasting because you like it. **NO**! You are going through the wilderness because, just slightly ahead, there is "*a promised land of weight loss and improved health that will take you to unprecedented levels of physical, mental and spiritual freedom*". I want you to **SEE** that promised land.

Say to yourself: *"Just for today, I will continue with the fast with eyes firmly-fixed on my health-improvement goals. I will spend time in my journal taking stock of my life. I will ask the God of my understanding to show me what I need to see and grant me the spirit of revelation. I believe that I am being healed physically, mentally and spiritually and am grateful for the beautiful gifts I am receiving through fasting".*

Day 6

We are now at **DAY SIX**! Regardless of how you may be feeling today, six days of fasting is an amazing accomplishment. **By now you have walked through the very worst of the fast and have confronted your human weaknesses in ways you may have never done before.** You will definitely walk away a much stronger and sharper person as a result of what you are doing.

At around day FIVE, roughly 80% of the "*surface*" toxins in the bloodstream and digestive system have been eliminated. So today you may be feeling "*a little*" better. But there is still another round of symptoms coming up. I want you to be ready. Around DAY SIX, the body starts to dig into the "*deep*" toxins that "*hide*" inside muscles and stored fat. These are the worst of the worst and, consequently, cause the harshest of the hunger pangs and detox symptoms.

This phase lasts until day 10 to day 14, at which point symptoms and hunger will diminish. Remember, some people may experience hunger and symptoms for as long as 21 days - depending on overall health and level of toxicity. If this is the case with you, **DO NOT BE DISCOURAGED**! It will pass, it will pass, and it will pass! Oh, and I forgot to tell you: it will pass! Hang in there... <u>you are well on your way</u>. You've come way too far to give up now! If you weigh yourself today, **it is probable that you may have lost as in excess of 10 pounds**. How much weight have you lost? Log it in the fasting journal. **The fastest daily average of weight loss happens over the initial 7 days of fasting.**

However, the fat burning machine continues. Even now, as you read this, your body is eating away stored fat and making you leaner and healthier! Weakness and dizziness usually linger. Sometimes these symptoms are such that one can hardly move. That is normal. Again, rest is the best way to handle it. If you can spend most of your time relaxing, reading, writing and maybe watching a few good movies; that would be best. Please <u>**DO NOT**</u> make any plans that require too much activity. Once more, I remind you to drink at least **ONE GALLON** of water daily. Log the frequency and quality of your bowel movements.

Are you still regular? Have the bowel movements decreased in frequency? Increased? **By day six of water fasting, it is possible that your trips to the toilet will be less frequent.** When you <u>DO</u> have a bowel movement, <u>do not be alarmed</u> if the stools dare darker than usual, almost black. That is **GOOD**. Your body is ridding itself of some very toxic and disease- causing debris! **If you have been constipated, then that reinforces the need for more water.** Did you call your **DESIGNATE** buddy and get active in a forum? I hope you did. The time for procrastination, second-guessing and doubting is over. Now is the time to believe, even if the mind tells you that all of this is poppycock. **We take action anyways.... <u>in spite of ourselves</u>**.

Do not lose sight of how much you have left of green tea, chamomile tea, seltzer, Valerian Root, etc. Promptly take stock of your supplies, identify what you may need from the store and go with your friend. You should definitely **<u>NOT</u>** go to the supermarket alone at this point. If it cannot be helped (*because no friends are available*), then the best way to do it is to blindly walk directly to the items that you need and promptly walk out. Do not linger in the store for any reason. Use *The Time Trap Escape*. You are becoming a real pro. I am proud of you!

Say to yourself: *"Just for today, I will revisit my journal entries from the last five days. I will ask the God of my understanding for strength to reach my goals and objectives. I am grateful for all I have learned and look forward to the rich blessings that fasting gives my mind, body and spirit. Just for today, I will have joy and happiness - realizing that the best days of my life lie ahead."*

Day 7

Good morning my dear friend: Congratulations. You are reaching the completion of an entire week of fasting! Great job, great job, great job... you are showing amazing resolve and power of decision. You are actually in the minority. Of the billions and billions of human beings on the phase of the earth, very few have accomplished seven full days of voluntary fasting. So I want you to pause for a moment, go stand in front of a mirror and pat yourself on the back saying: *"You've done well. I am proud of you and I believe in you."*

Go, do that now ... great! Most of us are very quick to chastise ourselves when we fall short, but rarely pause to complement when we reach a goal. I want you to realize the immensity of what you are doing; give yourself the credit that you deserve! Fasting is never easy. Yet you are still here. Well done!!! Now let us buckle down and continue the journey. Let's meditate on the warrior's mindset! Repeat out loud:

"This day, I make an unshakable commitment with myself to go all the way

and do whatever it takes to accomplish my goals! I will hang on for 30 days! I will hang on for 30 days! No matter what! No matter what! No matter what! I will not stop! I will hang on for 30 days! No matter what! No matter what! No matter what! I will not stop! Rain or shine, hunger or detox symptoms, I will hang on for 30 days! No matter what! No matter what! I will not stop!"

By **DAY SEVEN** most people are feeling better and better, although weakness and dizziness can be strong. As I have already said, be careful - move slowly, do not rise too quickly from a sitting position. In rare cases, some people experience fainting. The best way to prevent this is to get as much rest as possible. If you need to go somewhere, ask a friend or family member to drive you. Tread with much, much caution today. Rest, rest and more rest is recommended.

Again, if you are still experiencing strong hunger pangs and/or detox symptoms, just relax. As I mentioned before, green tea helps a lot to soothe symptoms and to give you a pep of energy. Use it as your shield. The same goes with seltzer water. But please make sure not to drink more than four bottles of seltzer water daily as it may irritate your stomach and cause more discomfort. Are you spending time in the journal and reaching out to your **DESIGNATE** buddy? Do not ignore or set aside this recommendation. It is very important to have somebody close to you who knows what you are doing and is in your corner. A 15-minute chat with a close friend who supports you will go a long ways in renewing your strength and allowing a wave of hunger to pass. We are going forward and making progress. But we have to remain very vigilant, as the mind is a cunning foe.

As always, drink as much water as possible during the day. Spend some time writing about what you are feeling physically and mentally, as well as any other insight, thoughts and/or ideas that may come your way. Writing on the journal constantly while fasting is *(by far)* one of the best ways to make it through those rough spots.

Remember: each moment of fasting awakens your spiritual side more and more... none of this that you are going through will be in vain. Keep your eyes on the prize; keep reminding yourself of your objective and do not let the mind focus your attention **ONLY** on "*how uncomfortable I feel*". You can do it! Keep at it and do **NOT** give up!

Say to yourself: "*Today I will remember my goals and not focus only on the discomfort. I will emphasize the huge positive health benefits that I am receiving through fasting. I will keep the vision of that "new me" on my mind. I will walk through whatever challenge comes my way. I thank the God of my understanding for the strength, grace and power to make it through these 24 hours of fasting*".

Day 8

Good morning: Congratulations on making it to another day. You are moving deeper and deeper into your land of miracles. How are you feeling? Are you sleeping well? Remember that you have the chamomile tea, tryptophan and valerian root to help settle you down at night so that you can sleep. If you find yourself feeling agitated during the day, take a tryptophan tablet and have a cup of chamomile tea. It will help to center you and give you breathing room to get through the immediate challenge. Let's refocus our minds and hearts with the *warrior's mindset!* **Repeat out loud***:*

"This day, I make an unshakable commitment with myself to go all the way and do whatever it takes to accomplish my goals! I will hang on for 30 days! I will hang on for 30 days! No matter what! No matter what! No matter what! I will not stop! I will hang on for 30 days! No matter what! No matter what! No matter what! I will not stop! Rain or shine, hunger or detox symptoms, I will hang on for 30 days! No matter what! No matter what! I will not stop!"

Today I want to start sharing with you a

system that helps me a lot whenever I am fasting. **How to R.E.A.C.H. My Goals**. I use the acronym R.E.A.C.H. to illustrate these 5 steps because that's your job as a water fasting practitioner ... **to reach and achieve the weight loss and health-improvement goals that you want.** To bring to reality the changes that will allow you to have the quality of life that you want. Is that not what you want? I am sure that it is. Here is how R.E.A.C.H expands:

R – RELEASE yourself from guilt and self-condemnation.

E – ENJOY life today -right here, right now.

A – AVOID sugar, starches, caffeine, fats & junk food of any kind.

C – CONSIDER the impact of what you are doing.

H – HANG on to your dreams and never back down.

There is a lot of power in those five points. Let's begin to look at them one by one.

Step 1: "R" RELEASE Yourself from Guilt & Self-Condemnation: On speaking to more than 50 people who started a long-term fast and failed - guess what the number one reason was for their fall? Yep -> <u>Guilt and Self-Condemnation</u>. *"I just did not feel I was worth all of this trouble,"* said Jim, 47, who has been 80 pounds overweight for five years and struggles with hypertension. *"I have always messed up. I have never done anything right when it comes to food. I had faith in failure; I did not believe I could lose the weight. All I constantly did was put myself down; I just couldn't stand the sight of myself,"* he said.

Sadly, this describes the mentality of many people that e-mail me. Can you relate? In which way do you find yourself caught in guilt and self-condemnation? Write about it in the journal. Get to know that voice that wants to bring you down, that wants to keep you from accomplishing your goals. When I get these emails, I always ask very important question:

What mistakes have you made that you keep putting yourself down for?

Answer that question in the journal to see what comes out. If you have tried fasting and/or dieting in the past and have failed, then it is highly probable that you *say negative things to yourself related to those unsuccessful attempts.* It is possible that being lean and healthy is a far-fetched ideal that, in your mind, you do not feel you deserve or are good enough to attain. Whatever the situation might have been ... whatever failures you may have had in the past ... no matter how many times you have tried it before and failed ... **TODAY IS A BRAND NEW DAY!** Let the past go!

"Visualize yourself dropping a box filled with the past into a bottomless pit. Gone! Forgive yourself for your mistakes! Continuously rehashing past mistakes will **NEVER** produce the positive change we are after in this course." One can fast for a hundred days. But the change will be fleeting if destructive mental patterns are not challenged. You already have started to confront the negativity. It is imperative that you rid yourself of guilt and self-condemnation. If your mind is full of *"what could have been but never was"* or *"what I have done to myself"* or *"the worthless or inferior person that I am,"* (*or any number of variations of this negativity*) – then you will **ALWAYS** find some reason to break the fast.

The mind will usually feed you some negativity like: *"why should I deserve to accomplish something that will make my life better?"*

Step 2 "E" ENVISION Yourself at the Ideal Weight / Health: Another top reason why people start a long-term fast and then break it prematurely is because *"they allow the mental negativity and detox symptoms to cloud their vision of what they want to accomplish."* An effective way to sidestep this common pitfall is to create a collage of body pictures that are in line with your goals and spend time daily looking at them – especially when you are fasting and struggling with hunger and/or detox symptoms. You told me that you were willing to do whatever it takes. So today I am going to take you at your word and ask you to do a little project.

Do this:

Browse through magazines and cut out pictures of sleek and fit bodies. **Note**: You can, of course, also do this by surfing the web and printing out the images. Cut the head out of a picture of yourself from some family album or other photograph. Paste it to the body picture image from the magazine. This worked great for me. Looking at my face in the thin body from the magazine kept me focused on what I wanted to accomplish.

Looking at that photo interrupted the negativity that urged me to give in.

It helped to snap away from the trap and press forward with my goals! Paste the pictures in *"trigger"* locations such as the bathroom mirror, the nightstand or desk right next to your bed (*so it is the last thing you see at night and the first image you intake upon awakening*), and - of course – the refrigerator door. Every morning when you get up look at it and tell yourself: "**This is me. This is how I want to look physically. I can do this.**" **Remember; nothing tastes as good as thin feels!**

Build a *"collage"* of fit bodies taking part in a variety of athletic and recreational activities and stick your head into the bodies. This *"envision"* step is a mighty weapon that you can place in your fasting arsenal. It is truly amazing. I realize that, for many, this whole thing about building a collage, pasting their face on fit bodies may seem silly and pointless. There's that voice again... talking down about the things that are given to you to help you. Ignore the voice, ignore *'feeling silly'* and do the exercise anyway. Trust me... it will help you a lot. You still have a ways to go and need all of the weapons that you can get. So get to work on the collage and we will continue with step 3 tomorrow.

Say to yourself: *"Today I am releasing all negativity and resistance. I becoming willing to completely let go of all thoughts that want to discourage me and cause me to fail. There is no failure for me today because I release all of it from my mind. I let it go completely and watch it as it leaves my life for good. Instead, today I am filled with passion, strength, commitment and determination. I cannot be moved because the Grace and peace of God is upon me... I am safe to continue in my path. And I can rejoice because, today... all is well."*

Day 9

Good morning my dear brother / sister. How are you feeling today? You are almost at double digits. That's the point of no return, you know? You are moving further and further into the process. Can there possibly be anything that could cause you to give up at this point? No way! You are locked in my friend. You are totally committed. You drew a line in the sand and separated the past from the future. And it is in this present that your new future is being created. By being willing to continue through this fasting path, and by facing the challenge, your entire destiny is being rewritten from inside your heart **OUT** to your body and the world. In that note, we again receive strength, hope and inspiration from the *warrior's mindset*. Recite aloud:

"This day, I make an unshakable commitment with myself to go all the way and do whatever it takes to accomplish my goals! I will hang on for 30 days! I will hang on for 30 days! No matter what! No matter what! No matter what! I will not stop! I will hang on for 30 days! No matter what! No matter what! No matter what! I will not stop!

Rain or shine, hunger or detox symptoms, I will hang on for 30 days! No matter what! No matter what! I will not stop!"

What you're doing is huge. You're willing to walk through discomfort and do things that you normally wouldn't do, all for the purpose of improving your life and health. That takes guts my friend! If a friend did all of that for you, would you not consider him or her special? Yes, of course. **The relationship with yourself, the most important of all, is also healing**. The more you move forward and stay the course, *the more you show to that man or woman in the mirror that you care for him or her.*

Let's continue to step 3 of the acronym R.E.A.C.H.

Step 3 "A" AVOID Sugar, Starches, Caffeine, Fats & All Junk Food. We have touched on this before; the need to make a firm decision that **NO LONGER** will you allow these foods to control you, harm your health and cause you to become overweight. No longer! Make a commitment with yourself **RIGHT HERE AND RIGHT NOW** that, once the fast is over, you will **NOT** return to these toxic and destructive foods. They were part of the past. However, they no longer serve any purpose in your life. You are aware of their allure and destructive power and are **NO LONGER** willing to give in to their subtle invitations. No more, no more, no more... that filth is **OUT** of your life for good. Of course, the implementation of this decision you are making is done *'one day at a time.'* Each day, when I wake up, I pray and ask the God of my understanding to help keep me away from that first bite of the junk foods that used to harm me. If I don't take the first bite, then I cannot binge and fall by the wayside. Today, I pass on this same willingness to you... will you take it?

Step 4 "C" CONSIDER the Impact of What You are Doing. This step challenges you to expand your fasting journal... to stop skimping on the surface and, instead, go deep into your heart and identify the impact of what you are doing. What have you been writing about in your journal? Have you written at all? Or have you scribbled a few *"quick thoughts"* without giving it any profound thought? I hope that has **NOT** been the case. If it has, then I want to give you a subtle nudge and ask you to do it!

NOW is the time to grasp this assignment and start to really dig into it with everything that you have! I have **NEVER** seen anybody complete a long-term fast that did not have clear, written reasons as to why they were doing it. Step 2 helps you to reinforce what you want to accomplish, visually. **This fourth step, however, is the most crucial of all because, with it, you are exploring your soul's deepest and fondest dreams.** You are digging into the very core of your existence to determine what you consider to be your heart-felt goals and ideals as these relate to health. *"Your dreams, hopes and ambitions must all be in writing so that you can see and read them."* Why? Because most *"fasters"* suffer from a very short memory, especially when amidst a long-term fast and stricken by hunger pains and detox symptoms. They seem to forget the heartbreak and devastation of even a week ago.

How they felt when on their last binge of overeating; when they looked at themselves in the mirror and saw the rolls of flab all over. The disgust and remorse of the past is forgotten. The mind, as usual, will attempt to *trap you in time* by erasing your long-term goals from memory. **It will persuade you to give up**. If you have nothing in writing that you can go to and remind yourself why you are doing what you are doing, then you'll be very vulnerable to the mind's subterfuges. This baffling mental assault caused me to fall many, many times.

Permanent change requires focused and consistent action.

I give you every weapon in the arsenal. But if you file the information and allow it to collect dust, then it will not do much good. You may not be prepared for the battle and could become a casualty. We have had enough of that, haven't we? Today, spend more time writing the '*reasons*' why you are doing this fast. Add detail... **heart-felt emotion and detail**. Spill your heart into the paper and hold nothing back. We are not doing this to be martyrs or masochists. Rather, we are doing it to improve the quality of our lives. **In short**: The words written in your journal ALONG with the visual stimulus from the Step 2 collage create a potent "*two-punch*" combination that will help you tremendously to counteract detox symptoms, hunger and negativity.

Day 10

You have broken into phase two of your water fast. Ten days is a <u>HUGE</u> accomplishment. Of the dozens and dozens of people that I have coached in the past five years, hardly any make it to ten days of fasting. They want to fast. They are honestly struggling and know they need to lose weight. But, for some reason, they are unable to muster the inner strength and determination to make it very far. So you, my friend, are an amazing person. I wish I could be there where you are so that I can literally huge you and tell you how proud I am of you. I mean it. We are together in this journey. Your breakthrough is my breakthrough because we are fellow travelers in the road of self-mastery. Isn't that what fasting is? Self-mastery? Yes.

And you are moving further and further into a powerful chasm of self-realization that will lead you to all of your dreams.

Keep going!

Step 5 "H" HANG on To Your Dreams and NEVER Back Down! This step won't work unless you have done steps two and four.

Here is where you are able to see why you are taking time from your life to do this fast and produce these changes in your life. Join me in a quick journey through time, space, the past, the present and future ...

Let us go deep into our hearts and minds and find the strength to overcome. Maybe you have tried it all before and have always gained the weight back. Perhaps you have tried every diet under the sun and nothing has worked. Maybe you are ill ...

...maybe you have very little hope that anything will ever work. But, then, when you start to write about your dreams and goals ... something happens inside of you. For a minute, even for just an instant, you start to believe that... maybe; just maybe... it is possible. You visualize yourself wearing that dress or pant-size that you always dreamed of. You think of wearing a bathing suit and feeling good about walking around on the beach ... proud of what you have accomplished...

... You no longer have to be ashamed or hide from the world. Or maybe you dream of a day when you will not feel sluggish and full of inertia and apathy towards life. You want to go up a flight of stairs without huffing and puffing ...

...you want to think clearly and be rid of the confusion and overall mental fatigue that plagues you. You want to look and feel better ... you want your life to be full of energy and health. You want to walk this earth and be the best that you possibly can ...

... You want to maximize your time here and give your family, your community and the world the very best of you... no matter what your role in life may be ... whether you are a parent, an employee, a manager, a director or an international mogul... you need your health, right? You want your world to be filled with optimism and hope

... So that when all is said and done you can, in your heart of hearts, have absolutely no regrets. You gave it your very best and had the courage to overcome your struggles. And the struggles themselves served to forge your character so that you could positively-influence the lives of everyone around you ...

... Amazing, huh? How the very struggle

that was there to bring us down eventually became our greatest asset ...

...These are many of the elements that make up life... that make up destiny and fate. And they are all in your hands – right here, right now. The fork in the road is before you. The two paths are clearly made and in your sights. Which will it be? Will you give up and continue to go through life thinking about *"what could have been?"* Or are you going to press on and reach the goals?

...Put the past behind you. Forget about all of your failures and disappointments. We have all had them. Today marks a brand new beginning. The slate is clean and the sky is the limit. This is the first day of the rest of your life...

...Believe ... believe, my friend, that you are worth it. Believe that you can reach **ALL** of your dreams and goals. Do not allow your mind, people or the world tell you – even for a minute – that you are finished or that you are not strong enough to make it...

...They are lies, lies ... all lies! **YOU CAN MAKE IT!** And you are worth it! This is the moment of truth ... the moment where a brand new destiny is being written for you by the universe...

... And you are now walking the road-less-traveled of **CHANGE** that will take you where you always dreamed... there are no more limits... no more impossibilities. You are free!"

Day 11

You are now on day 11, one step closer to the goal. Have you weighed yourself? How much weight have you lost? The goal is 30 pounds, but - as I said before - you very well could lose even more. It all depends on how your body responds. This is the final motivational message. However, there is plenty of '*meat*' in all of them to keep you going until the end of the fast. Please return to the message from day 1 tomorrow and make your way through them once again. Apply the suggestions that I give you with greater emphasis this time around. Whatever you may have skipped the first time around, now you have the opportunity to do it again.

This is what I call "**The Next Phase of Development**." This basically represents the rest of your life. The collection of 24-hours that will depict your existence from today forward. Which way will it go? Will you persist with the principles you have learned and accomplish/retain your freedom? What will determine what the coming years will be like for you? That's what this fast is all about. And, of course, you have all of the *masterclass* content, which I want you to continue to listen to and study, day and night while you are fasting. Some people tell me they even go to sleep with the *masterclass* on their *iPod*. Use the material in whatever way you find most useful, but use it! My message to you today is this:

FREEDOM CARRIES SACRIFICE

This is particularly true when it comes to weight loss, body cleansing and changing eating habits. I am sure that by this point you know exactly what I'm talking about. Hunger and detox symptoms are always looming and beckoning you to give up. At least that is the case with me. I am not "*cured*." For the past ten years I have not relapsed into binging and I have successfully kept myself at a trim 200 pounds. But I have had to sacrifice. I don't mean sacrifice in a morbid or ascetic way. What I mean is that I have had to realize that, if I wanted to protect my weight and health, I had to realize that I was not "*just like everyone else*." The crowd eats mindlessly and pays little or no attention to future health consequences. The crowd wants - the crowd eats. The crowd craves - the crowd gives in. That is the status quo and the way in which millions live their lives. But that is **NOT** what you have learned here. You must separate yourself from "*the crowd*" and treat yourself with the unique respect and delicate-kindness that you deserve. Your choices in food from now on can **NEVER** be the same.

You have awakened from your slumber and can no longer be counted in the sleeping masses.

You want to be lean, healthy and vibrant. And it is your desire to accomplish/maintain this not "*just for a little while*," but for life - right? Yes, it is! **Say to yourself:** "*Today I surrender completely to this fast, mind, body and spirit. I open my heart and mind to receive the strength and power of God, which fills me with infinite power, wisdom and supernatural determination. Nothing can stop me because I have let go of all the negative. I may hear it and feel it, but I no longer react to it. All negativity MUST yield to my spiritual determination. I believe that the light of God inside of me burns through all negativity and* *destroys every behavior, habit or belief system that leads me away from my goals. I am renewed in mind, body and spirit and am filled with peace. I am loved. I am safe. I am free!"*

Chapter 19

Ending the Fast

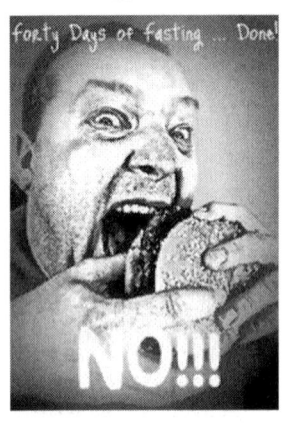

Breaking a fast is the most important part of the process, right? Yes, I've said that to you like four times already. I'm sure you're sick of hearing me say it. But it is absolutely true. I have run into many people who fast for thirty days and more... but they break it inappropriately. This is unwise and dangerous.

The digestive system has been inactive, so we have to wake it up slowly and steadily. You can literally place your life in danger if you do not break a fast adequately. One man that wrote me said he fasted for 14 days and broke it with a cheeseburger. He got horribly ill and his stomach swelled up like a balloon. Like me, he nearly ruptured his stomach lining and died. I was heartbroken for him. Well intentioned... but not properly informed. So we must tread carefully. Not only that, but I also want you to come face-to-face with hunger and **NOT** give in to it. **Hunger comes back strong when one first breaks a fast**. The key is to stick to the schedule I have outlined.

Do not "*hurry*" things because you "*think*" that you are ready. I have fallen prey to that mental trickery and can tell you that it is **NO FUN**. It takes hard work to complete a 30-day fast. There is nothing more discouraging than to give away the benefits at the last moment. That is like the man whose boat sinks and he is forced to swim for days in the cold, dark ocean. Finally, he sees the beach up ahead but, just as he is about to touch land, he decides to stop swimming and sink to the bottom. What! All of what swimming for nothing? No way! **Here's my point: The stricter you are with the process of breaking a fast, the greater the benefits and the stronger your foundation will be for long-term**

success.

Chapter 20
Weight Gain After Fasting

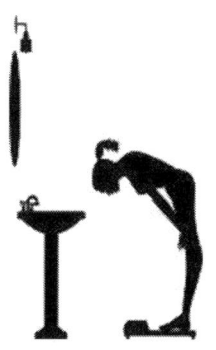

No matter how closely you observe the re-feeding regimen, breaking a fast always leads to weight gain of 5-10 pounds in the first 14 to 21 days. This is no reason to freak out, as many do. The weight gain is a totally normal reaction to a long-term fast. The body was in ketosis for a long time. This is basically the body's starvation/survival mode.

During the fast, the body scavenged the body in search of anything it could devour (*autophagy*), eating pure fat on a daily basis. When you break the fast, the body, still alarmed from the fast, begins to 'hoard' energy *'just in case'* another survival situation happens (**the body doesn't know that you were fasting intentionally**).

In addition, while fasting the metabolism slows down considerably. When you couple the body's exit from starvation mode and a sluggish metabolism, the result is the weight gain I've described. <u>AND</u>, we cannot forget that at the point of breaking a fast there will also be a certain amount of water weight gain. **All of this is normal.** There is no reason to be upset. What matters is that you **continue to eat a clean diet with portion control**.

Over the following weeks, if you keep eating clean and healthy, then you will find that you are starting to lose the initial weight that was gained. Fasting produces very fast weight loss. That means that, after fasting, your body size is likely quite smaller than it was when you began. The body needs time to get used to this new order of things. Don't obsess on scales and numbers. Instead, go to the nearest sports shop and purchase a device to **measure body fat**. Rather than the scale, start to rely more and more on your body fat level. That will give you a much more precise verdict of where you are. I had times when the scale said I weighed four pounds more, but my body fat levels had actually decreased! As you can see, pounds can be deceiving. But body fat measurements don't lie and are always constant. Plus, scales cause many of us to get way too emotional. And that often leads to discouragement and the *'screw it'* syndrome. But you have come way too far to succumb to any screw it syndrome. Bottom line: The initial weight gain observed after breaking a long fast will be shed once more over the coming months, **IF** you keep a clean, portion-controlled diet (*more about that later*).

Chapter 21
Post Fasting Shopping List

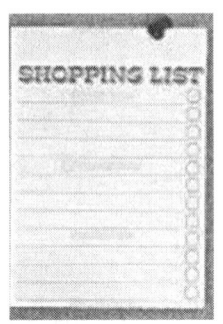

Ok, it is time to break the fast, and there are several items that we need. First and foremost you are going to need a juicer. Most people already have one. If you do not, you can usually find them at your local discount store for as little as $20. If you can afford it, I'd suggest that you get a good and sturdy one. Please do not disregard this requirement and break the fast with just any juice. I want you to roll up your sleeves and prepare it from whole fruits and veggies. That's where the real power is! Once you have the hardware, then it's time to get the produce. During the last few days of your fast, go to the market and pick up some supplies. **Here's my personal "breaking a fast" fruit/veggie combination:**

* Apples – One Bag
* Pears   Five or Six
* Oranges – One Bag
* Celery – One Bag
* Carrots – One Bag
* Spinach –One Bag
* Cucumbers – Three or Four
* Watercress – One Bag

Your body will receive a tremendous jolt of nutrition. Of course if you have a personal juicing recipe, go ahead and use it. But make sure that you combine **BOTH** fruits and vegetables. Set aside at least two apples and two pears for **eating only**. Don't juice them. We will need them as part of the re-feeding process. Also from the produce section, get some lettuce, tomatoes and a couple of lemons. In addition to the produce, you'll need a bottle of Probiotics to help repopulate the *'good bacteria'* in your stomach. Check in the dairy section to see if you find Kefir. Unlike yogurt which contains transient bacteria that do not repopulate the digestive tract, Kefir has active, growing and *'living bacteria'*. This is a marvelous boost to your system, and will swiftly repopulate the digestive tract.

Moreover, get some chicken broth packets, some low-fat milk, a bag of flax seeds, a small bottle of olive oil and a package of some good oat bran cereal (*not the sugar-filled commercial type please!*). These items can usually be found at the health-food section of many supermarkets. If not, then you can order them online. I have added some Amazon.com links above for your convenience. Amazon, in my experience, is cheap and fast. Finally, purchase a bottle of some natural juice. I use grape and orange, but you can choose whatever type you like best, even vegetable juice. **Keep it simple**. A good juice from the health-food section in your local supermarket will more than suffice.

After day three you'll prepare your own juice by liquefying fruits and vegetables with a juicer

For starters, a good bottled NATURAL JUICE is enough, so long as its sugar content isn't too high. Shoot for a juice with 15 grams of sugar or less. Do NOT, by any means, use a juice that is high in sugar as that would defeat the purpose of what we're doing. Check around and read labels until you find a juice that fits the bill. If you are unable to find any juice that is low on sugar, then purchase the best one that you can and dilute it 50% with water. I do that with orange juice all of the time. I love **OJ**, but 25 to 34 grams of sugar is obscenely high; the only way I can enjoy it is by diluting it with water. We have to be extra careful because we're breaking a 30-day water fast and everything that you eat and drink must be closely monitored. Alright, that is the end of the shopping list! Please make sure to have these items in place **prior to the last day of your fast**. Do not wait until the last moment. Now let's look at your daily re-feeding schedule. *Re-feeding is what I call the process of starting to eat after a period of fasting.* When you are ready to break the fast, start with the following chapter.

Chapter 22

Breaking the Fast (10-Day Guide)

Re-Feeding: Day 1

Upon arising, drink two large glasses of water. Over the next hour, meditate on all that has transpired over the course of your fast. Take some final notes in your fasting journal. Talk about how you are feeling mentally, physically, emotionally, etc. If you practice a specific religion, pray and "*turn over*" the fast to the God of your understanding. You have done A LOT of work. You have shown courage, steadfastness and faith. Once you feel satisfied with your prayer/meditation/journaling time, break the fast with an eight-to-twelve-ounce glass of watered-down juice. NOTE: This is a very powerful moment. Do not drink the juice nonchalantly. What you have done has great significance for you, your future and for your loved ones. Make sure you drink the juice sitting down and with a thankful and prayerful heart. Some people like to gather their immediate family and have a small celebration. I have photos of me ending one of my first long water fasts, and I'm surrounded by immediate family, distant relatives and even a priest (*that I'd never met in my life*). Seriously, completing a 30-day water fast is a tremendous accomplishment. You are one of the few on this planet who will taste the delights that fasting always gives those who have the courage to walk through the tempest.

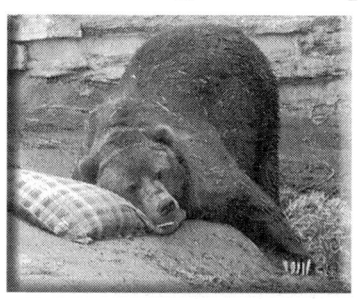

Drink the watered-down juice. One glass only please! Remember: the digestive system has been dormant (*like the sleeping bear above!*) and needs to be roused **VERY SLOWLY**. You don't want to make the bear angry, do you? **NO**... believe me, you do <u>NOT</u> want to startle the bear!

Wait TWO hours and drink another glass of watered-down juice. Drink two more glasses of water. You should feel no irritation or discomfort. If you do, then you will need to dilute the juice even more. To keep it safe, I suggest you mix it 50-50.

Continue to drink a glass every three-to-four hours for the rest of the day. Make sure to consume at the very least half a gallon of water throughout the day. Keep a fasting journal close and write any thoughts and feelings you may have. The first few days of breaking a fast are filled with deep introspection and insight. Make sure to take the personal time to do just that. Good job! This brings to conclusion your first day of breaking the fast.

Re-Feeding: Day 2

Upon arising, immediately drink two large glasses of water (*I recommend you adopt this as a lifetime practice*). Again spend some time in your journal writing your thoughts, ideas and feelings. Write about how you are feeling physically. You may start to sense greater hunger at this point. It is important to remain vigilant. The mind may attempt to "*convince you*" that you are fine and can go straight to solid food. Don't do it! We want to lay the strongest foundation possible, remember? **For breakfast, drink an eight-to-twelve-**

ounce glass of your watered-down juice. Today, however, you can reduce the water content by 25%. Stir it well. Drink it slowly. Drink another glass in three-to-four hours.

If, three hours later, you feel **ZERO** discomfort or irritation, you can start to drink the juice without watering it down. Again, you should not feel any abdominal pain or irritation. If so, then return to the 50-50 dilution for another twelve hours. I can give you detailed instructions, but it is crucial that you listen to your own body and use common sense. Better to dilute the juice for another half day than to take risks. **Please listen to your body and proceed with much caution.** If all goes well, you will have finished the day drinking pure juice. Your digestive system will definitely start to reawaken. Ok! This brings to conclusion your second day of breaking a fast.

Re-Feeding: Day 3 –Juicing

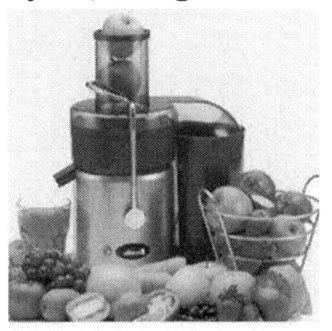

Upon arising, drink two large glasses of water. For breakfast drink a glass of your juice, and then take some time to prepare the juicing mix. If you are already experienced using a juicer, then proceed with the preparation instructions below. If not, then let me take a moment to acquaint you. Most juicers have a *primary pouring spout* that releases the juice extracted from the fruits and vegetables.

Some more expensive models capture the juice in their own compartment for later pouring. If you have the former, then you will need an *8-to-12-ounce glass* to place underneath the spout to capture the liquid as it comes out. Moreover, you will need a *one-gallon jug* to store and refrigerate the juice. We will also need *aluminum foil* to wrap the jug and protect the juice from the light in the refrigerator which can prematurely spoil the precious liquid. I know that sounds silly since the fridge is usually closed and dark. But I actually have had juice spoil prematurely and it is very disheartening. So stick with me. I won't lead you wrong, I promise! Another section of the juicer that I want you to notice is the *"waste"* compartment where the pulp from the fruits and vegetables is discharged. Do you see it? I recommend that, for easier cleaning and disposal, you place a plastic bag (*I use small supermarket bags*) inside this partition as one would put a bag inside a trash can. That way all you have to do when you're done is remove the bag, close it and discard the leftovers. **Vegetable and fruit pulp spoils rapidly and can create a foul odor.**

<u>Note</u>: There is really nothing *"wasteful"* about pulp, however. It has huge amounts of fiber and some of it is even tasty. We are actually going to scoop some of the pulp and mix it with the juice to help with bowel movements and detoxification! If you are unsure about where the pulp compartment is located in your juicer, refer to the

instructions manual of the model that you purchased. Assembly is finalized by snapping in place the top cover over the liquefying blades. This cover normally includes the vertical feed opening where the produce is inserted. Once the top snaps into place, you will then be left with a plastic or wooden *"pusher tool"* that is used **to press the fruit and/or vegetable down the feed and into the grinder for liquefaction**. Take a moment and review the parts I have just mentioned.

Get acquainted with your juicer. By all means, make sure to read <u>ALL</u> of the instructions that came with your hardware. If you just purchased it, make sure to wash each part thoroughly with soap and water <u>prior</u> to assembly. This is important. A juicer I purchased years ago, upon close inspection, had rotten chunks of fruit and vegetable on the cover and blades. Apparently it had been used, returned and nobody bothered to clean it. It was just dropped back in the shelf for purchase. Gross! Clean, clean, clean that juicer very thoroughly before you do anything else. Once the juicer is ready and you have become familiar with how it works, then it is time to set it in place. Find the place in your kitchen counter where you intend to put the juicer. Find the largest possible area near an electric outlet. Now place a large towel (_or two_) to cover that entire area, placing the juicer on top of the towels. Using those towels will help a lot to minimize the mess. In addition, some of the darker-colored fruits may stain your counter. Make sure that the towel(s) cover the entire counter area where you will be juicing.

Prepping the Produce

Take the fruits and vegetables out of the refrigerator and place them on the kitchen counter. For now, leave them in the containers (_or bags_) in which you purchased them. Do this as close to the sink as possible. Take out two bowls and set them aside. Also take out a cutting board and sharp knife for dicing and peeling. If you have a fruit/vegetable peeler, then use that. **Now we are ready to start prepping the produce for juicing. Let's take them one by one**:

* **Apples** – Take three out of the bag, wash them very thoroughly and cut them in half. Remove the seeds from the middle and place them in the bowl. Do not peel away the skin from the apples as it will create some good pulp!

* **Pears** – Take three out of the bag, wash them very thoroughly and cut them in half. Remove the seeds from the middle and place them in the bowl. Do not peel away the skin from the pears as it will create some good pulp!

* **Oranges** – Take two oranges, wash, peel and cut them in half. Place the four halves in the bowl.

* **Celery** – Rip four sticks of celery from the stalk and wash them thoroughly with warm water. Celery stalks often contain traces of dirt in them. Once they are clean, place them in one of the bowls.

* **Carrots** – Take three out of the bag. Shred the top layer of skin from each carrot by holding it diagonally in the sink and running the knife horizontally from top to bottom as a scraper. You can also use a potato peeler. Once the carrots have been scraped, wash them thoroughly in warm water and place them in the bowl

* **Cucumbers** – Wash thoroughly, peel and cut in halves
* **Watercress** – Rinse a medium hand full and set it on the bowl.
* **Spinach** –Pick a handful from inside the bag, rinse under warm water and place in bowl for juicing.

Once you are done with the peeling and cutting, you will have an amazing site in front of you: **a bowl overflowing with beautiful fruits and vegetables ready to enter and cleanse your body!** Look at the bowl for a minute and ponder at the wonderful benefit that you are about to receive. Let the site fill you with the vision of health and weight loss that you have for your life.

I realize that getting to this point required some work. You may have never done anything like this before. You might even have had to overcome apathy, depression and/or discouragement (*among others*) to get up and actually take the action. My first time juicing was not a very joyous occasion. It took a **LOT** of push to make myself do it because I was so disgusted with my weight and health. Maybe you have been ill. Maybe you have tried many different paths and nothing has worked. Yet <u>you are here</u>. You have shown willingness. Congratulations! Keep it up! I feel proud and honored to have you with me!

The Pusher or 'Guiding' Tool

We are now ready to juice the fruits and vegetables. There really is no order or science as to how you should juice. I juice fruits and vegetables in random order as I grab them from the bowl. The best way to start is with celery which is by far the vegetable with the most juice. From there you can simply continue with whatever fruit or vegetable is in front of you. About the *"pusher or guiding tool."* As I mentioned earlier, most juicers come with a plastic or wooden tool that is used to guide the fruits and or vegetables into the feeder. **It is very important that you know how to use it properly or you will reduce the yield of juice**. We do not want to waste any of this precious juice!

<u>**DO NOT**</u> push down on the tool! Once you insert a piece of produce into the feeder, allow it to go down at its own pace. Simply

use the tool to *guide* the fruit or vegetable down to the grinder. **DO NOT FORCE IT DOWN!**

The **MORE TIME** each piece of produce takes to make it down the feeder and into the blades, the **MORE JUICE** you will get. Use the pushing tool as a guide and do not force it!

Always Remember: **MORE TIME = MORE JUICE**.

In some cases, as with cauliflower or broccoli stems, you may need to push *lightly* to ease the stress on the juicer blades. The same can sometimes happen with oranges, pumpkin and carrots. But, for the most part, you should <u>minimize the pressure</u> you exert on this tool.

Allow the fruit or vegetable to make it through the feed on its own as much as possible.

Use the guiding tool to follow the produce down the feed, but push down on it only when necessary.

The Juicing Process

So, when you are ready:

Place the 8-to-10-ounce glass under the

juicer spout to collect the liquid. Be sure to place some napkins or paper towels underneath the glass to absorb any spillage. Turn on the juicer and let it warm up for twenty seconds. Then, take the first piece of celery and put it into the feeder. It will start grinding and bouncing around, getting smaller and smaller until it disappears into the blades. Observe the light green juice coming out of the spout and into the glass. Now let's try a chunk of apple. Insert it into the feeder and follow it with the guiding tool into the blades.

Depending on the size of the opening, you may need to cut the apple into smaller pieces. With apples, you won't get as much juice as you did with the celery, but watch it come out. Get used to the different color liquid that goes with each fruit and vegetable. The juice you are seeing come out are fruits and vegetables in their purest form! It is life, weight loss, healing ... optimum health, mental clarity, detoxification, energy ... it is, in essence, <u>your own personal fountain of youth</u>. Let these thoughts enter your mind as you continue the juicing process. At this point simply move on to the next fruit or vegetable in the bowl and repeat the process. As I said, carrots, pumpkin, oranges and broccoli may need a little push down. For leafy produce like watercress, sprinkle little bunches into the feeder. You will see the little spurts of dark green juice coming out of the spout and into the glass. Whenever you see that the glass is getting full, turn off the juicer and pour the liquid into the one-gallon jug you purchased. I put a funnel on top to avoid spillage. But, **MAKE SURE** that you have an empty glass to place under the spout immediately as some juice will continue to ooze out **even after the juicer is turned off**. We want to capture that also! Then turn the juicer back on and continue the process. Continue emptying the contents of the 8-ounce glass into the jug as it fills, always turning off the juicer and putting the *"backup"* glass under the spout to capture any dripping.

Pay close attention and do not allow any of the juice to spill! Inevitably there will always be some spillage, but it should be minor. <u>**DO NOT**</u> juice while you are *multitasking* - talking on the phone, watching television, or when otherwise being interrupted or distracted. This is a precious and *sacred* time for you and it should be treated as such! Focus on what you are doing! Once you have completely juiced all of the produce into the bowl, turn off the juicer and observe the *fruits* of your labor. If you used a half-gallon jug, it should be almost full, or halfway if you utilized a gallon container. I never get tired of just looking at the multi-colored liquid as it sits in the container. Now that is pure power!

Adding the Pulp

Let the juice breathe uncovered for a few minutes. Unsnap the top of the juicer and direct your attention to the *waste* or pulp compartment. You will see the *pasty* leftovers of the fruits and vegetables. **That is far from garbage**. It is pure fiber which is great for the belly! Scoop two tablespoons of pulp and dump them into the juice. **You may want to eat a few spoonfuls. I love it.** Now, remove the plastic bag from the pulp compartment and zip it closed. I recommend that you **DO NOT** let this bag sit with your kitchen trash. Take it outside until garbage day. Some people who enjoy gardening actually use it as fertilizer. I am not a gardener and have never tried this. But I have heard it works very well.

Cleaning the Juicer

Now it is time for what probably is the least enjoyable part of the process: <u>cleaning the juicer</u>. Leave the juice uncovered and turn your attention to disassembling the juicer and placing its parts in the sink. Most juicers come with a small brush for cleaning. Make sure to unplug the juicer before you start disassembling it! You can probably rinse most of it off, but it is **VERY IMPORTANT** that you spend as much time as needed **brushing the blades and removing every last trace of pulp**. When you are done, the blades should look as though they were never used! Do not cut corners. Dirty blades lose their sharpness quicker, and **even small traces of pulp can rot and contaminate any juices you prepare in the future.**

Wipe down the main juicer, ensuring that all traces of juice have been cleaned. When you are satisfied the cleaning has been thorough, set the juicer parts aside to dry.

Finish the cleaning process by removing the towel from the kitchen counter, wiping off any spillage and grinding any fruit or vegetable skin (*that you peeled earlier*) in your garbage disposal. Follow this system every time you juice. **It is best to clean right away while you are giving the juice time to breathe.** That way, when the time comes to drink, you can do so in peace without having to worry about doing any cleaning.

Handling & Tasting the Juice

During the cleanup process, you set the juice aside to breathe. Now, screw the lid tightly on the jug. Make sure that it is tight and that no juice will spill. Then turn it upside down and shake it vigorously for about 30 seconds. It is amazing to see the pulp mix with the rest of the juice, leaving a layer of foam at the top.

At this point, if the jug is not completely full, you can cap it with more water and the vegetable juice you purchased. But don't add too much vegetable juice. One glass of water and one glass of vegetable juice should be more than enough to fill the gallon jug nearly to the top. If not, that is fine. You've done a great job. Now to the best part of all ... drinking the juice! Fill a glass with the juice and have a taste! Drink it slowly, visualizing the powerful healing nutrients entering your bloodstream and digestive system – cleaning and wiping out toxins in their path! Most people love the taste of the juice. If you do not, then don't worry about it. It will grow on you. The next time you juice, you can start to add a bit more or less of certain produce.

Eventually, you will find the taste that works best for you. But this is not about focusing on the taste. Watercress tends to be bitter, especially if you have never had it before. Or some other unusual taste may stand out. Give it time and focus on the benefits that you are gaining in weight loss and health. If you have spent years eating a lot of unhealthy junk, then this is truly a gourmet feast that your body is **VERY** thankful to receive. Now, screw the lid tightly on the jug again.

Take out the aluminum foil and cover the entire jug as if you were wrapping a present. What better gift to your life than this, right?

Once sealed, place the jug in the refrigerator. It is best to place it in a spacious location where the jug doesn't have to be constantly moved to access other items in the refrigerator. We want the juice to be protected and secure at all times. If there are young children at home, I suggest that you instruct them not to handle the jug on their own as they may drop it or otherwise spill it. But, by all means, give them a taste! If you can get them used to drinking pure fruits and veggies when they're still young, you will be giving them one of the best gifts that they could receive. **By mid-to-late afternoon you should have finished preparing the juice**. Fill up an eight-to-twelve-ounce glass and sit down in the kitchen table, or wherever you are. This juice will take you to the next level because it contains much more sustenance, fiber, pulp and nutrients than the juice you drank the first two days.

Take a break of at least 10-to-15 minutes and enjoy the juice. It will taste like heaven, trust me. *Drink it slowly and savor the pulp as it hits your tongue.* Chew and savor it as this powerhouse of nutrients goes down your throat to your eagerly-awaiting belly. What a glorious moment! You completed your fast, and now you are celebrating by breaking it slowly and honoring your body for all of the cleansing, weight loss and healing that it has done. **Thank your body for its loyalty, even at times when you mistreated it**. Make a covenant with yourself that <u>NO MORE</u>... from this day forward you will eat and live healthy... even if that means going against what others are doing. *You are on the road less traveled.* You are on the road to a much better and vibrant life. If so moved, take out your journal and write whatever comes to your mind. Spend some time in contemplation, listening to that internal *Voice*... that gentle, small Voice in your belly that wants to give you direction, revelation, knowledge and deep insight. Pay attention! This *Voice* is speaking.... even now as you read this! Make sure to refrigerate and cover the juice so that no light enters because it can spoil it prematurely.

In another three-to-four hours you can drink another glass of the juice. At night, make sure *not to drink after 10pm*. If you are awake and hungry, drink two large glasses of water or crack open a seltzer. A cup of soothing chamomile tea will also help. Remember, as the digestive system reawakens, so does the hunger monster. So **you have to be extremely careful and vigilant**. If you are new to fasting, then you may not have been eating all that great. Old habits, behaviors and belief systems will attempt to regain control of your life. They will try to enslave you once more. Do **NOT** allow it! Stay alert and focused! Yes, the fast is over. But this is not the time to lower your guard. Food cravings are cunning and will always look for ways to make you fall. If you can accept that reality, then your chances for long-term success will be much greater. Congratulations! That concludes your third day of breaking a fast.

Re-Feeding: Day 4

Upon arising, immediately drink two large glasses of water. Some people have a watery bowel movement the morning of the fourth post-fasting day. If you do, then that is a clear sign that the digestive system has resumed its duties. But don't worry if you don't; more than likely it won't happen for another day or two. **At your usual breakfast time, go to the refrigerator and take out the jug of juice you prepared yesterday.** Shake it vigorously so that the pulp mixes in well. Making sure that the lid is safely in place, turn the jug upside down and shake it some more. Pour yourself a glass and sit down to drink. Look at the contents and observe the colors and small particles of pulp floating around. You are looking at pure nutrition and health, amazing huh? Continue to take this morning time to write in your journal, recording how you are feeling physically and mentally. If you have any spiritual readings that you are accustomed to doing, then by all means do so. **For the rest of the day, drink a glass of juice every three-to four hours, not exceeding 64 ounces or "8" eight-ounce glasses.** *No juice should be drunk after 10pm at night.* In the measure that you drink the juice, pour water into the jug to replenish. We don't want to water it down too much.

However, if you are careful, adding some water will "*stretch*" the yield for up to four and even five days. Another good way to extend the yield is to add some veggie juice into the jug. Some people ask me if it is okay to add ice to the juice. The answer is **YES**, but do it sparingly. Do NOT turn the juice into a frozen beverage please! You should not feel any discomfort or irritation. For hunger, increase your water consumption and rely on seltzer and tea. You are doing a great job. Make sure to get plenty of sleep and do not overexert yourself physically. **The body is getting stronger, but it still needs some time.** This concludes day four of breaking a fast.

Re-Feeding: Day 5

Upon arising, immediately drink two large glasses of water. You may or may not have a bowel movement at this point. Today we are ready to move to yet another phase of breaking the fast. At your usual breakfast time, go to the refrigerator and take out **ONE** apple and **ONE** pear. Cut the fruit into four slices each, pour yourself a glass of water and sit down to eat. One apple and one pear is more than enough initially. Chew slowly and wash the fruit down with lots of water. This is your first real "*solid*" food, so it will taste like the nectar of the gods! Enjoy it... you worked hard and deserve it! **Wait EIGHT hours.**

Sit down and eat another plate of fruit as you did earlier. Today you can drink juice every TWO hours. So utilize it to hold you up during the day when hunger strikes. Make sure to continue to drink at least half a gallon of water daily throughout the process. The digestive system will thank you for it! If you are accustomed to going to the gym or taking part in some type of physical activity, today you can resume, albeit at a reduced capacity. **You will likely find yourself struggling with hunger.** Just drink lots of water and seltzer. DO NOT give in to the desire to eat more than what is allowed. I want you to receive maximum benefit from your efforts. Breaking the fast slowly and steadily is very effective. Do not eat or drink any more juice after 10pm. That is more than enough for today. Goodnight!

Re-Feeding: Day 6

Upon arising, immediately drink two large glasses of water. In the majority of cases, you will have a bowel movement at some point today. If not, you certainly will by tomorrow. For breakfast, take out an apple or pear (*whatever you like most*) and cut it into small pieces. Go to the cupboard and grab the oat bran cereal you purchased. Measure out **ONE** cup and pour it into a bowl. Add **ONE** cup of low-fat milk. Sprinkle the fruit on top. Sit down to eat! This is yet another phase. Now we are giving the digestive system some oats and bran... which will help immensely. Again, the hunger will want you to inhale the cereal. Don't! **Eat slowly, taking care to chew the food up to 30 times before swallowing.** When you are done eating, take one Probiotics capsule. How are you feeling? This is the most you have eaten since you broke the fast! Is the food going down smooth? Any pains, aches in the belly? You should not have any. If you do, then go back one day and eat fruit only for another 24 hours. If all is well, you can eat one apple and one pear in eight hours and drink a glass of juice every two hours - just like yesterday. By the end of the day, the juice should pretty much be gone. Great job!

At dinnertime (no later than 8pm), take out the lettuce, cucumbers and

tomatoes and make yourself a salad. We don't want this salad to be **HUGE**, so don't eat with your eyes. *Half a head of lettuce, a cucumber and a tomato will more than suffice.* For dressing, add a tiny amount of olive oil and a squeeze of lemon. Mix it well. Sit down to eat with a large glass of water. **Again, eat slowly and chew each bite until it dissolves in your mouth.** Take your time and enjoy. Drink a full glass of water when done. Great job! If you get hungry for the rest of the night, drink more water and/or seltzer. How about a cup of soothing chamomile tea? Allow at least two hours after eating before you go to bed. If you can go for a short walk, that would be terrific. Have a good night!

Re-Feeding: Day 7
Upon arising, immediately drink two large glasses of water. Today is going to be EXACTLY like yesterday, including the Probiotics in the morning after your cereal. At around 2 or 3pm, however, mix a heaping tablespoon of flax seed into an eight or twelve ounce glass of water or juice. Drink it! Eat your salad at night and make sure to continue to drink lots of water. For certain,

your bowels will be moving. When you go, it should be easy and effortless... no straining. Those are the amazing benefits of a super clean digestive system! Excellent. That's it for today.

Re-Feeding: Day 8

Upon arising, drink two glasses of water. Today will be exactly like yesterday. Cereal, fruit and low-fat milk in the morning with your Probiotics and flax seed mixed with water or juice in the afternoon. At night, however, make yourself a cup of chicken broth. **INSTEAD** of the usual salad, today you can also have steamed vegetables in small quantities. (*I like broccoli, carrots, squash and cauliflower*). You are allowed small sprinkles of olive oil, salt and parmesan cheese for either the salad or veggies. **The broth and veggies are the largest meal to date!** Eat slowly and chew well. **DO NOT** gorge! Seriously, I have known people who break long fasts with huge plates of vegetables marinated with olive oil and salt. That's sheer insanity. It's not just about what you are eating; it also has a lot to do with quantity. When breaking a fast, it is best <u>NOT</u> to bombard the system with large amounts of food – even if it is vegetables. Eat, but take it easy. Again, you MUST resist the desire to overeat. If you get careless, you will pay for it with physical and emotional discomfort. So **PLEASE** (*pretty please!*) be careful. That concludes day eight of breaking an extended water fast.

Re-Feeding: Day 9

Upon arising, immediately drink two large glasses of water. Today will be exactly like yesterday. Oat bran cereal in the morning with sliced fruit and low-fat milk. Probiotics. More fruit during the day accompanied by flax seed beverage in the afternoon, and your broth and salad (*or veggies*) at night.

Re-Feeding: Day 10

On the TENTH day after the fast, start with your usual glasses of water, oat bran cereal and fruit. Now it's time to go to the market and stock up for the Phase II STANDARD DIET. Yes, that means that you finally get to eat a little more. But if you followed the last nine days as I instructed, you have protected your fasting efforts like a lioness would her little cubs. This is what has to be done. Slow is fast, remember? Yes, if you take each step slowly and with a clear structure, the risk of relapse is notably lessened. And, after all, that is what we want, correct?

<u>A note of warning</u>: *Here is where many people fall off the wagon and start to backslide with their diet. The hunger will be notable since, even though you broke the fast, you still are eating substantially less than you normally would. So the physical hunger is normal, and so are mood swings and irritability.*

Have you ever seen how mad Fred Flintstone would get when he was hungry? Yes, you might even growl. So what? Growl away... but **DO NOT** give in! This is a very important transition. To do it properly it must be carried out with great caution, and follow the specific menu that I'm about to give you... ok? While I use countless diet combinations, below is one that helped me to break 25 years of obesity and binge eating. I completed a 40-day water fast, did the ten-day re-feeding **EXACTLY** as described above, and then switched to this. So I am going to make it ultra-easy for you by simply telling you what do to and expecting it to be carried out exactly as instructed. I told you I would give you direct instructions, and that is what we are going to do here. Right now, let's look at the simple diet you will follow from now on!

Chapter 23
The Permanent Weight Loss Diet

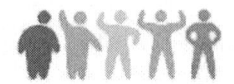

Now it's time to go shopping, to begin the amazing journey of transforming your eating habits with a structured diet that I call *The Permanent Weight Loss Diet*. Why do I call it so? Because, in my experience, as long as you follow it to the best of your ability, the diet will help you lose weight as well as maintain. In other words, this diet has helped me to lose weight and **KEEP IT OFF**!

And the beauty is that you will get to eat plenty; good, clean foods that will nourish your mind and body. After a few weeks of observing this diet, you will feel terrific. First I am going to give you the shopping list. I actually gave you a lot of this information earlier in the *pre-fast preparation chapter*. However, I am going to include it here again so you don't have to keep scrolling back and forth to find it. At any rate, the information is relevant in both the pre-fasting preparation and the long-term diet structure that we are looking at now. So, as I was saying, we will look at the menu in detail, and - *after that* - I will give you tips on how to prepare the meals as quickly and easily as possible. As I said at the start of the book, the best way to lose weight and keep it off is to have an eating structure. And yes... that means that you will be cooking for yourself.

Even if you have a loved one who is willing to cook for you, I strongly encourage you to start by doing it yourself. The food preparation process, over the course of weeks, will impact you very positively. You will begin to see that you **CAN** maintain a clean diet. Cooking my own meals is something that gave me a great deal of self-esteem and satisfaction. What was even more amazing was when the pounds started to drop off. Having abused food for so long, it was hard to believe that I actually was not only cooking, but cooking meals that were good for me! That was a **HUGE** departure from being locked in my apartment for weeks, without bathing or shaving and constantly ordering pizzas and Chinese food. This was different. This was **me doing good things for me**. Perhaps for you cooking isn't a big deal. That's great. You're way ahead of the game. But most overweight people that I talk to tell me that they only know how to cook junk. One lady actually broke down in tears when she first started to cook for herself. "I can't believe I'm actually taking care of myself... being responsible for my health," she said. "What about you? Are you ready to start taking care of yourself? Yes, I believe that you are. In the past I was a slave to whatever other people were cooking.

Or I was a slave to my own apathy and laziness, which would lead me to eat the worst foods possible, "*because I hate cooking.*" But let me assure you. When I talk about cooking, I don't mean that you will be expected to prepare complicated meals. The diet is very simple. Basic cooking is all that will be required. Ok, enough yapping. The shopping list and menus bellow were already presented in the *Cleaning Up Your Act* chapter. However, to make it easier to navigate through the book (*so you don't have to keep going back for the info*), I decided to include them here as well.

Chapter 24

Shopping List

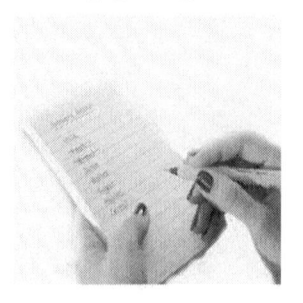

* **Boneless Chicken Breast** - Try to find a bag with six or ten breasts, I often go to the freezers and grab a large back of breasts from there. You need to have your protein, so stock up on the chicken.

* **Extra Lean Ground Turkey Breast** (*no deli turkey*). Ground turkey has been my saving grace, let me tell you. I was so confused and whacked out of my mind when I first started doing this, that even cooking a piece of chicken on the skillet was difficult. Ground turkey is very easy to cook, can be mixed into eggs for breakfast... and it basically is my lifeline. When buying ground turkey, but the one with the least amount of fat please. Don't just grab the first serving you come across. Stop and read the labels... find out how much fat it contains. I would say that a package of ground turkey that is 85% meat, 15% fat should be fine. You can drain the excess fat later. The 'fat-free' ground turkey can get quite expensive and, to be honest, it tastes like the sole of a shoe. It is very tough, dry and not very tasty at all. Stick to the 85/15 for now.

* **Egg Whites;** Yes, real eggs are out. We want the protein from the egg whites, but not the fat and cholesterol from the yolk. I had a real hard time letting go of eggs because I ate them almost daily since I was a toddler. I loved eggs, but I had some form of asthma or allergic condition, so I was not allowed to eat eggs. I would still eat them, however. Even if I had to get up while everyone was sleeping, I **WOULD** eat eggs! As you can see, my tendency toward rebellion, wanting to do things *'my way,'* and disregarding council were alive and well inside of me. So no eggs please. Egg whites are fine. I have gotten used to them and no longer obsess over real eggs like I used to. **Note**: I use the liquid egg whites that come in a box because all I have to do is pour into the pan and cook. Besides, I always make a huge mess separating the yolk! :-)

* **Low Sodium Tuna Fish <u>Note</u>**: This kind usually can be found in envelopes rather than cans. You're going to be getting your sodium directly from the foods that you will eat. No salt is to be added to any food at any time for any reason. That's not cause for you to give up and throw in the towel, is it? Right now, we are barely getting started. We need to lay a strong foundation, and that includes foods that you must avoid. But that is no surprise to you. You know what you have to do. I'm here as your guide and facilitator... as your coach. But you and you alone are the one that needs to keep walking forward.

* **Fresh Fish** (*Tilapia and Grouper. Salmon Once Weekly <u>ONLY</u>*) - Fish can be expensive, so what I do is I buy it frozen from the supermarket refrigerators. Most markets have a decent variety of frozen fish. Tilapia is great and very lean. Grouper would also do the trick. You don't have to fill an entire cart with fish, but by all means pick up a few bags. Of course if you can afford to buy wild, fresh fish... then that is definitely the way to go. Farm fish give me the creeps, to be honest. Those fish are given all kinds of

pesticides. Many are even given artificial colors. Yes, if the fish is orange... the orange was man-made. The fish itself did not acquire that color on its own.

* **Baked Potatoes** -are my saviors. I just love them. I can come in from the street famished and all I have to do is nuke one of those puppies for ten minutes and it's good to go.

* **Sweet Potatoes** - I love sweet potatoes as well. Very easy to prepare. Potatoes and sweet potatoes are good starches... complex carbohydrates that will give you clean energy. There are potatoes that come wrapped up in plastic ready to be tossed into the microwave. While that IS very handy, these supermarkets want like $2 for each. Just on principle, I won't pay it. Maybe where you live these pre-wrapped potatoes are cheaper.

* **Quaker Oats** (*100% Whole Grain, Quick Oats*). Another complex carb that I rely on every day - especially in the mornings. Get a good amount.

* **Cream of Wheat** (*White Box*) Get a good amount as well so that you can mix these up

in your breakfasts.

* **Cream of Rice** - all great stuff, awesome complex carbs rich in fiber... clean food that will cleanse and transform your body.

* **Pasta** (*Only Whole Grain or Whole Wheat - No Egg Noodles*) I'm a pasta freak. So the rule of thumb is to stick <u>ONLY</u> to whole grain or whole wheat. Anything that is enriched (white pasta) should be deemed garbage and not consumed.

* **Brown Rice** - I love my brown rice, especially the boil-in-the -bag type which requires no cooking. I am terrible cooking rice, that's the truth. It nearly always comes out mangled and chewy... a total freak show. So I stick with the boil-in-the-bag, and it works very well.

* **Fresh Green Vegetables** (*Broccoli, Carrots, Cauliflower* etc...) **<u>Note</u>**: These are great for steaming. I usually purchase the bags that come with them already pre-mixed.

You will find a lot of different veggie combinations to choose from in these pre-mixed bag selections. I like these because all I have to do is wash them and steam them.

Again... keeping it simple, right?

* **Balsamic Vinegar and Olive Oil:** These two are going to be your salad dressing from now on. All other dressings are banned. Most of them are packed with sugar and fat. Do **NOT** add any dressing other than the olive oil and balsamic vinegar. I was a *Blue Cheese* nut. I'd eat it every day... I'd put Blue Cheese on my cereal if you let me. Well, not really... but you get the idea. When I was first confronted with having to stop using it, I kicked and screamed. I admit it. I had a hard time using only olive oil and balsamic vinegar. However, today I wouldn't trade them for anything in the world. I look at a bottle of blue cheese now and it sickens me that I was eating all of that fat and sugar.

* **Garlic and Onion Powder** -Ok, these are the puppies here that you will use to spice the food. But you have to make sure that you get the garlic and onion powder, **NOT** the garlic or onion salt. In addition, pick up a few bottles of **Mrs. Dash No Salt All-Purpose Seasoning.** Those three are basically the only seasonings that I have used in many years. I no longer add salt to anything. There are different kinds of *Mrs.*

Dash. Pick the one you like the most. I like the Garlic & Herbs mixed with the garlic and onion powder. They come together very well and do the job. I don't miss salt at all. Give it time and you'll get to the same point, trust me.

*** Enrico's No Salt-No Fat Spaghetti Sauce** (*Or Any Other No-Salt Brand You Find*) Alright, this Enrico's sauce is very good. However, it is often a pain in the neck to find. Go to the pasta aisle in your local supermarket. If you don't see it there, see if they have a *'specialty pasta'* display anywhere in that vicinity. If not, they may have it in another aisle under *'heath foods.'* Ask a supermarket clerk for assistance. Tell him or her that you need a pasta sauce that comes with **NO SALT ADDED**. If they don't have Enrico's, he or she may direct you to another brand. Just make sure that the pasta sauce has no salt added.

*** Stevia Sweetener** (*No Equal or Splenda*) I realize that you may want to have a cup of coffee or tea in the morning, or that you may want to sweeten up the oatmeal. I mean, who wants to eat oatmeal plain, right? Might as well eat a piece of cardboard. Yes, we're going to go with the Stevia sweetener, By **NO MEANS** do I ever want you to consume Equal or Splenda. I'm not going to get into that speech right now. Suffice it to say that I don't want you to put any toxins in your body. And those artificial sweeteners are toxic and harmful. Stevia is alright... it is a leaf. It does tend to have a slight bitter under taste. So at first you may be cursing me from afar when you use it. But in a few weeks you'll totally get used to it.

* **Any Sugar-Free and Low-Sodium Salad Dressing** - Going back to dressings real quick, I had forgotten that there **ARE** some brands out there that come with no salt or sugar added.

If you take some time and peruse the displays, I'm sure you will find something that will work. Ask the supermarket clerk for help. It took me about an hour to find my *Olde Cape Cod Raspberry Light* dressing. Look for that same on where you live and see if you can live with it. It is the one with the lowest amount of salt and sugar that I found

* **Fresh Strawberries or Cantaloupe** -

Good stuff. We are cutting out refined sugar, but natural sugar from fruits (in moderation) will be just fine. Strawberries and cantaloupe are two of the fruits with the least amount of sugar.

* **Hunts No Salt Ketchup** (*If you like ketchup*) Maybe you don't eat ketchup. I, on the other hand, have been on ketchup since I was a toddler. But I only use it occasionally, and I stick to the no salt kind.

* **Gilda Toasted Bread** (*no salt or sugar added*) - These toasts are great to kill the hunger in between meals when used sparingly. They can usually be found in the bread or health-food aisle of most supermarkets. I can't tell you how many times a Gilda toast has saved me from disaster. We need to be ready because we know that the body will be complaining a lot, and the mind will be trying to harass you - talk you into giving up. We know that it is going to happen. The difference is that we are preparing. We will be ready. **YOU** will be ready.

* **Seltzer Water (Sparkling Water/Club Soda)** - If you have visited my website FitnessThroughFasting.com and read some

of the content, you may have heard me mention seltzer water. Years ago, while I was in the middle of some very tough hunger pangs and detox symptoms, a friend of mine just casually said "Here, drink this." The moment the effervescence hit my stomach, it was like magic. The hunger calmed down almost right away and the symptoms became much more tolerable. I'm telling you, seltzer is the bomb. It is a crucial weapon to have in our arsenal, so make sure to stock up with a 24-pack at least.

* **Decaffeinated Green Tea** - Green tea is yet another weapon that we want to have in our arsenal. Green tea has body-heating properties which help to give you a pep of energy as well as accelerate weight loss. I am not putting all of my bank on the 'weight loss' aspect of the tea. It is true that it has body-heating properties. And when we are dieting, hungry and weak, we need an ally such as this to come and restore us.

***Decaffeinated Coffee** - I mention 'decaf' here because, in my process, I decided that I wanted to be free of all stimulants, including caffeine. I always ended up drinking more than I should, I'd get all jittery and end up succumbing to a food temptation mostly because of frustration and irritability. I would prefer if you joined me and let go of all stimulants as well. It may seem like an impossible request at first, but today... I don't miss coffee one bit. And I was a massive coffee drinker. Obviously I cannot force you to stop drinking coffee if that is what you wish to do. But I **CAN** tell you that as long as you have stimulants in your body, the risk will always be present that something could set you off and lead you to do something foolish.

***Chamomile Tea** (*To help soothe nighttime hunger and help in case of insomnia*). This tea is absolutely magnificent. I rely on it to help settle me down at night. I'm a nighttime person, so many times I have a hard time turning in at a decent hour. As we talked about earlier, when we are dieting, a lot of toxins are released into the bloodstream while the body detoxifies. Sometimes, this release of toxins can cause insomnia, a sense of mania or, as it happened to me, nightmares. Chamomile helps to pretty much neutralize all of that unpleasantness so that I can lay down and get some rest.

* **Valerian Root** (*To Help You Sleep*) Here's another excellent herbal supplement. This sucker works. It knocks me out every time. Take one or two tablets if you are having trouble sleeping.

***Tryptophan** (*This is an amino acid that also acts as a mood stabilizer and could help you sleep at night if you find yourself restless*) But a bottle of the 500 mg tablets. Tryptophan has a very calming effect. Sometimes when dieting, we may get really frazzled about a situation, or we may simply fall into a very foul mood. We may wish to lash out at "the other people who can eat and I have to stick to this BS structure." When I get into those dark spaces, taking one tablet of Tryptophan can help to calm me and give me the window I need to escape from the onslaught.

Chapter 25

Smart Eating

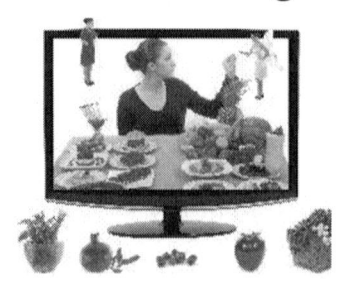

That's it! When I first give this list to personal coaching clients, they ask me if somehow I made a mistake and gave them too much food. Yes, this is a good amount of food, right? Even today, I am amazed when I walk to the kitchen table with this plate packed with meat, pasta, salad and veggies.

This is good eating. This is what the body deserves. And even with all of this food, you are going to lose weight. The whole point is **NOT** to **NOT** eat, but rather to **EAT SMART**.

I want you to be as comfortable as possible and, even more, I want you to be able to get through your daily schedule without dragging your elbows on the ground. You still are going to feel the pinch, don't get me wrong. This is a very solid fat-burning diet, so you will have moments when hunger and other symptoms will come around to holler at you. But whatever you go through will be tolerable because you are eating good amounts of clean, healthy food.

Let's finalize the shopping list by making sure that we are **<u>CRYSTAL CLEAR</u>** which foods are banned and which should be limited.

Chapter 26

Banned Foods

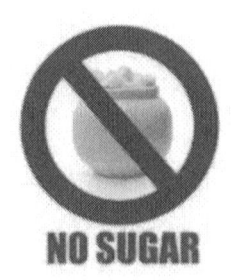

*Salt - you get plenty of it from the foods that you will eat. When I first started my diet years ago, I was kind of shocked to see that salt was banned. I spoke against it actually. I have come to realize that the foods we eat all have sodium, and that a healthy adult really has no need for 'salt' except to make the food taste better. In addition, when I stopped using salt, I immediately dropped like 15 pounds. It was mostly water weight, but it showed me that I was retaining a LOT of liquids, and that was greatly due to my abuse of salt and seasonings.

* **Sugar** - absolute trash, toxic to the body... good for nothing - stay away! I could write pages and pages about sugar. I am sure that you yourself can admit that this is one of our greatest (*if not our greatest*) enemy. I mean it. Enemy. Any prolonged return to sugar will, sooner or later, result in a full-blown relapse and the regaining of the weight that I've lost, I don't kid myself by thinking that "*I'm cured.*" I still am susceptible to sugar and to binging. What keeps me free is not to put sugar into my body... period. I can't draw the same conclusion for you, but I am certain that you probably have your own stories to tell about sugar and how it has affected your weight, life and health.

* **Fried Foods** - Absolute filthy grease fest that leads to obesity and other diseases.

* **Cheese** - Cheese is great but it has way too much fat. For the time being, steer clear.

Later on, once you reach your weight loss goal, you will be able to have treats from time to time. So don't let the mind start telling you that your 'life is over' because you can't eat this or that. Just tell the mind to shut up and keep moving forward. Works like a charm for me.

* **Dairy Products** - dairy has a lot of fat, is high in sugar content and has been known

to cause digestive system inflammation. But I'm not totally heartless. Stock to non-fat milk, how's that? Anything above non-fat is banned.

* **Red Meat** - I personally don't have anything against red meat. In fact, I have been known to eat a piece of meat on rare occasion. Right now, we are banning it because it has a lot of fat, and because I want your digestive system to be given easy food to digest. Later on you can have a piece of meat here and there if you want. Right now... it's banned.

* **Alcohol** - Alcohol is packed with empty calories. Calories with <u>ZERO</u> nutritional value. And booze turns to sugar. Bad all over. If you drink frequently, cut it down to a minimum. You're doing this for your health and to reach a goal that is important to <u>YOU</u>. If you have to go a few months without drinking, your arm is not going to fall off. You'll live. A cup of wine with dinner is fine, but nothing more than that at this juncture.

* **Butter or Margarine** - As they say in New York, "Forget about it!!!" Butter and margarine are pure fat and we don't want it.

* **Fruit Juices** - If you read the label of most orange juice brands, you will see that the sugar content is through the roof. Yes, it is natural sugar, but sugar nonetheless. You can have one glass of juice in the morning, but you need to water it down 50/50. Drinking straight juice at this phase is basically like injecting blubber directly into your belly. Stay away. Drink veggie juice instead...but make sure that it is the low sodium veggie juice.

***White Enriched Bread** - That stuff is like dropping a ball of cement into the stomach. That white flour, doughy garbage really is terrible for human health. I was going to ban all breads, but I remembered that the *Ezekiel* brand (*green bag*) is actually very good. You can eat one slice here and there as partial replacement to your carbohydrate servings. We'll get into all of that in just a minute.

***Junk Food of ANY Kind** - I think that it definitely goes without saying that junk food is out. And not just out for a little while.

Hopefully, it is out of your life for good. That crap is like wearing a ball and chain. It enslaves us to cravings that are never satisfied and only get stronger and more violent.

Foods to Limit List:

*Fruits (Stick To Strawberries or Cantaloupe)

* Tomatoes

* Peas or Corn

* Olive Oil

Take Immediate Action

So there you go. Take this list to the supermarket and fill it as soon as possible. **Today would be swell**. We have to move quickly and put you on this healthy eating structure; it's very important that you find your own *'pace'* and start making progress.

Go fill the shopping list and come back when you're done so we can talk about implementing the daily meal plan. I suggest that you take a friend with you to the supermarket, for support. You have cut out junk from your diet and are probably hungry.

So it's important to have somebody there

that can hold your hand and keep you from going crazy. We certainly don't want this trip to the store to turn into a binging debacle. So protect yourself and take someone with you to keep you in check.

One More Item: We are going to work on portion control. Therefore, you will need a kitchen scale to weigh some of the foods that you're going to eat. I suggest that you get a digital scale with large numbers for easy viewing.

Get one that weights in ounces since that is the measuring system that I will be using in the meal structure below. I have owned the My Weigh KD-7000 digital scale for several years and I love it. It runs around $40 and reads in grams, ounces, pounds and kilograms. If you don't already have a scale, please make sure to get one.

Chapter 27

Diet Implementation

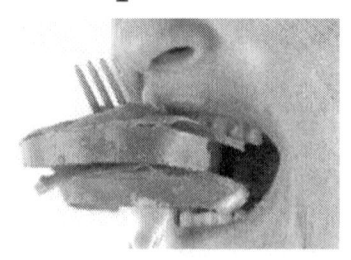

Ok, you have purchased all of the groceries needed for the diet as well as the scale, right. Now we have are ready to get into the implementation. How are you feeling? I want to make this process as easy as possible for you. Therefore, rather than putting together a menu based on what I normally eat, I have actually done something better. I've put together a chart for males, and another one for females. Simply follow the directions on the corresponding one and you're on your way.

This structure is effective because **YOU** can pick yourself what you want to eat (*based on the food groups and allowed portions*). This makes it **MUCH** easier because all you have to do is stick to the correct quantities of each food group ... period. In my opinion, diets **that try to make one eat this or that**

usually don't work because we are individuals with our own tastes and preferences. So this diet aims to give you as much flexibility as possible to eat what you like, and eat **A LOT**! The most important part of this process is to stick to the allowed foods and quantities. Alright? Let's check it out and get going.

Note: The meal structures below are based on a '*daytime*' schedule. However, I realize that many people may have a schedule that starts in the afternoon or even at night. That is fine. **Follow the meal times based on your actual schedule**. For example, if you work swing shift and don't get up until around *11:00AM*, you can have your breakfast meal at noon, and move forward from there. What I'm saying is this: make this diet **YOURS**. Use it based on **YOUR** schedule and the realities of your daily life. It will work just fine. The most important part is to stick to the food types and quantities and **NEVER** touch anything that is on the list of banned foods.

Serving Sizes

Protein Serving Sizes

Egg Whites 4-5

Turkey Breast 4 oz.

(<u>NOT</u> Deli Meat)

Chicken Breast 4oz.

Fish 5-6 oz.

(Limit Salmon and Shellfish)

Tuna Fish 4-5 oz.

(Low Sodium)

Carb Serving Sizes

Baked Potato 3-4 oz.

Oatmeal - 1/2 cup

(Dry Weight)

(Quaker Oats Only)

Sweet Potato 5-6 oz.

Cream of Wheat 1-2 oz.

Cream of Rice 1-2 oz.

Pasta - 1-1.5 oz.

(Dry Weight)

Brown Rice-

½ -3/4 cups (Cooked)

Gilda Toast 2 Slices

Meal Plan

REDUCE BODY FAT & CLEANSE
MALE:

*Breakfast: Start -> 8AM

2 Servings of Protein

1-2 Servings of Carbohydrates

*Lunch: 4 Hours -> Noon

2 Servings of Protein

1-2 Servings of Carbohydrates

*Afternoon: 4 Hours -> 4PM

2 Servings of Protein

1 Serving of Carbohydrates

*Dinner: Finish -> 8PM

2 Servings of Protein

Eat NOTHING else until breakfast next day for 12 hours daily of fasting.

REDUCE BODY FAT & CLEANSE
FEMALE:

*Breakfast: Start -> 8AM

1 Servings of Protein

1 Serving of Carbohydrates

*Lunch: 4 Hours -> Noon

1 Serving(s) of Protein

1 Serving of Carbohydrates

*Afternoon: 4 Hours -> 4PM

1 Servings of Protein

1 Serving of Carbohydrates

*Dinner: Finish -> 8PM

1 Servings of Protein

Eat NOTHING else until breakfast next day for 12 hours daily of fasting.

Chapter 28

Additional Instructions

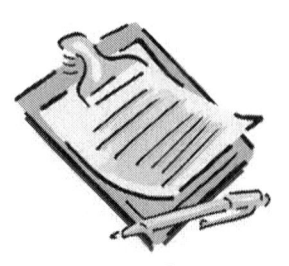

All measurements equal one serving.

Pasta: Use No Salt Spaghetti Sauce or No Salt Salsa. Steer clear of parmesan cheese, salt or any other seasoning apart from the ones in the shopping list (*Mrs. Dash, garlic powder, onion powder etc.*)

Vegetables & Salad: Fresh green vegetables and green salads can be eaten at any and in all meals. <u>NO</u> canned vegetables. <u>NO</u> bottled salad dressings aside from the low-sodium low-sugar ones in the shopping list. You can also use balsamic vinegar and/or fresh lemon juice.

Beverages: You may drink water, unsweetened tea, decaffeinated coffee (you can use the 'half-caffeine' type to ease detox symptoms) and seltzer water (sparkling water, club soda). Moreover, you are allowed one eight-ounce glass of non-fat milk daily. You can have the milk in your oatmeal, coffee or as a stand-alone glass at night before going to bed.

Food Preparation

Now let me share with you some tips on food preparation and the diet in general. You can make the dinner salad as large as you want it. The rest of the meals are to be followed <u>exactly</u> as written. Drink only water with the meals. Normally, an advanced cleansing diet would cut out even the meat. However, for the purposes of initial preparation this combination works very well.

If You're a Vegetarian

If you're a vegetarian, you can replace the poultry and fish with **plant-sourced protein in small quantities**. The best choices are well-cooked whole grain and bean combinations. The smaller the bean, the easier it is to digest.

Mung beans are well-known for their cleansing and protective attributes. Whole mung beans can be sprouted and eaten like a vegetable.

Brown rice and red lentils are another good protein combination. My personal favorite is tofu.

Nuts and seeds also provide protein but are high in fat and best eaten fresh in <u>very small quantities</u> (1/4 cup). With these variations, you will have no trouble completing the cleansing diet as a vegetarian.

Seasoning Fish & Poultry

Seasoning the Fish and/or Chicken: Make sure the fish or chicken pieces have been thoroughly washed. Squeeze fresh lemon on both sides of the meat.

Then you can add the customary garlic and onion powder and/or *Mrs. Dash* salt-free seasoning. When at the supermarket, spend some time in the seasoning products aisle and pick out your choice of the salt-free alternatives. A final option is to add a very light touch of apple cider vinegar for additional taste.

'Ziplocking' Portions

To expedite the food preparation process, I recommend that you pre-season enough meat (fish, chicken and ground turkey) for 7 days' worth of meals. Put the 6 or 8 oz portions in small zip lock bags. I keep enough meat in the fridge to last me around three days and freeze the rest.

I love *ziplocking (not a real word, I made it up)* because it gives the meat time to fully marinate. Also, it frees up my time because I don't have to go through the cutting, weighing and seasoning process every single day. Cutting, weighing, seasoning and bagging enough meat for seven days usually takes me around 25 minutes. Once it's done... You're good for an entire week.

To eat, all you have to do is pull out one of the baggies from the fridge and toss the meat on the pan to cook. I put labels on the zip lock bags and write in the exact weight *(digital kitchen scales are awesome)* as well as the date in which the meat was bagged. Dating the meat is practical because you want to make sure that older bags are always used first.

Every morning after breakfast, I take a few baggies from the freezer and move them to the fridge to cover my meals for another day or two. Simple tips, but they make the meal preparation process **A LOT** easier.

Cooking the Meat

To Cook the Meat: Spray a light coat of canola Spam spray on a cooking pan. Spam is the only kind of oil that you will be using during this cleansing diet. Turn the stove to medium heat. Place the meat on the pan. Allow it to brown on both sides with the pan partially covered.

A 6-to-8-ounce piece of lean fish or poultry should not take more than 15 minutes to fully cook on both sides. You want to make sure the meat is cooked thoroughly so as to ensure that all bacteria are destroyed.

About Caffeine

If you are an avid coffee drinker as I was, then eliminating this beverage from your diet completely will be a challenge during the next two to four days. You will experience marked headaches and probably be in an overall cranky mood. **Caffeine is a drug**.

I suggest that, if the headaches become unbearable, make a <u>small amount</u> of very watered down coffee and drink it to soothe. Do it first thing in the morning if that is when you usually drink the most coffee. **My**

headaches were massive and this helped a lot. During the day, what worked for me best was to carry some aspirin or other pain reliever and take a few tablets when the pain struck. See your pharmacist and ask for a recommendation that is best for you. Withdrawal from caffeine is a very important part of this detox process, so I encourage you to do it!

I am not telling you to give up coffee for good. That is up to you, although I do believe you would be better off to do so, or at least keep its consumption to a bare minimum. I was a coffee fanatic. Yet, once I got used to drinking non-caffeinated tea, I felt better than ever and did not miss coffee at all. The good news is that withdrawal from caffeine does not usually last longer than three days and the headaches will soon go away.

Chapter 29

Expected Weight Loss

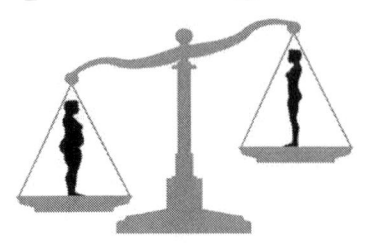

This eating structure will help you to lose anywhere from 10 to 15 pounds per month (*or more*). The diet is simple and comprised of common foods that I'm sure you are familiar with. How much weight you lose exactly will depend on your body's reaction. Ten pounds per month is typical, although I have heard of some that have lost 25 and even 30 pounds in one month.

Keep your expectations realistic and move forward with determination.

You **WILL** lose weight. In some cases, the weight loss is slow at first. But it picks up as the weeks go by. Such was the case with me. I lost 14 pounds the first month (*which is still awesome*). The second month I lost 20 pounds, and then the monthly weight loss stabilized at 10-12 pounds. I was very excited because I saw that, with the proper structure, anyone could lose lots of weight fast. And I have some good news. This is not a typical *'diet'* that starves the living daylights out of you and expects you to do it long-term while whistling and tap dancing. I don't believe in that because it simply isn't realistic. We all have jobs, families and schedules to keep.

So we need a diet that produces results, but doesn't cause us to walk around like zombies. I tried that extreme approach many times. And, given, occasionally one may choose to do a fast or some other type of ultra-restrictive short-term calorie restriction. Here, my aim is to give you a long-term eating structure that will help you to lose weight consistently.

And you still get to eat lots of great food and in handsome quantities. I'm not by any means saying that this will be *'easy.'* It will be *'easier'* than perhaps you would expect. But it still will require lots of commitment and willingness to walk through hunger and discomfort. The up side is that your body will get used to it after a few weeks. And, to be sure, the benefits in physical and mental health (*and weight loss*) will totally outweigh the discomfort. So I implore you to follow my instructions to the letter.

Let me be blunt: The initial phase of any weight loss program is hardest and the one that comes with the most physical and mental discomfort. But you're coming into this diet after finishing a 30-day water fast. So, while it may be challenging, this diet is certainly nothing that you can't handle.

All that I'm asking is that you put aside excuses and justifications and just stick to the plan.

I implore you to hang on and give yourself wholeheartedly to the task.

And that task, without a doubt, is learning to handle your stomach's demands; learning how to eat and overcoming the hunger barrier.

Chapter 30

Going Past the Hunger Barrier

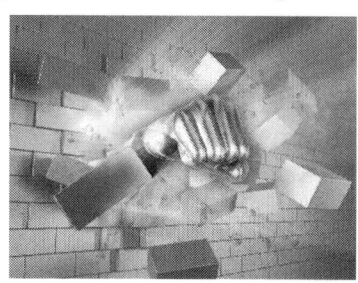

You have some experience with fasting, so you are probably not a stranger to hunger pangs and other symptoms. However, once the fast is over and you begin a standard diet, you will find yourself face-to-face with a new series of challenges. Keep in mind:

You are stepping into uncharted waters and beginning a deep physical, mental and emotional transformation.

Many people ask me: What can I expect to go through while on this standard diet?

You will likely feel hungry most of the time, initially

You will likely get angry and frustrated initially because you can't eat more

You may initially find yourself mentally planning a binge

You will likely be moody initially

You will likely become impatient initially because 'this isn't happening fast enough'

You may initially find yourself rationalizing 'why you can't do this right now.'

You'll likely initially find plausible arguments to justify giving up and eating whatever you want

You will likely get sick of cooking initially

You will initially crave the very foods you have eliminated from your diet

You may initially forget why you are doing this in the first place (to achieve permanent weight loss and health)

You may initially convince yourself that you would rather regain all of the weight and try later than to continue. "I just want to eat what I want, when I want it!"

You may initially feel sad and want to cry

You may initially dream about food

Believe it or not, this is all perfectly normal and **WILL** pass; the hunger will lessen over time as you get used to eating clean, healthy foods. Furthermore, you will be developing key mental and physical tools that will help you to master food and hunger, instead of the other way around. Positive change is never easy, especially when we confront negative patterns that have been with us for years.

One thing is certain: Positive change may be difficult (*initially*), but it is **ALWAYS** worthwhile. When you make it to the other side and experience that amazing sense of freedom and wellbeing, the sacrifices that you endured along the way will seem small and insignificant.

Right now, make a commitment with yourself that, no matter what, you are going to stick it out and adopt this diet into your lifestyle.

The key word in all of this is '*initially.*' Yes, initially it may be a pain in the neck, especially if, like me, you were a disorganized eater. But it gets easier over time and, before you know it, you are enjoying it and, even better, you're feeling clean, light, energized and vibrant. These are all benefits that I've received time and again from **The Permanent Weight Loss Diet.** And I hope that you come to receive them as well!

Chapter 31

The Battle of the Mind

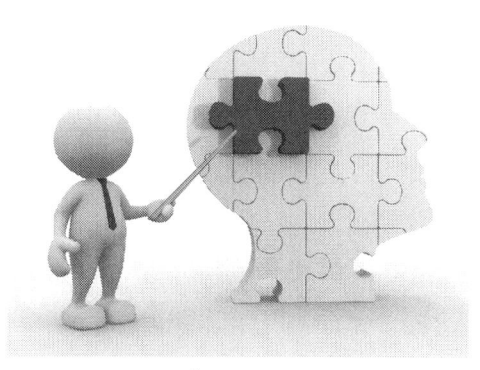

We have covered a **HUGE** amount of ground. You should be proud of yourself. I made it a point to throw in the kitchen's sink in this book so that you could have everything that you needed to succeed. Below is a listing of the action steps you will be taking to complete this work.

First, however, I want to leave you with a message: The **TRUE** victory over weight, food and overeating has nothing to do with food. It is all in the mind; our thoughts, belief systems and corresponding actions. A person with a *'fat'* mental picture of him or herself will have a very hard time staying thin, regardless of which diet they use. To that end, I want to challenge you to dig deep with your journal and write about **the things that you believe about yourself**. Here's an example from one of my old journals:

"I think that I'm a fat, ugly, loser that women want nothing to do with. I'm a fat, bumbling, awkward and uninteresting piece of garbage."

Can you believe that I wrote that in my journal right after I had lost 100 pounds and reached my goal weight of 195? I certainly wasn't *'fat'* then. But, amazingly, I continued to *'see myself'* as fat, ugly, unattractive and on and on. Realizing that I was going to regain the weight if I didn't change my thoughts and belief systems about myself, I launched an aggressive reprogramming offensive. You can read more about that in my other book, <u>How to Lose Weight & Keep it Off By Reprogramming the Subconscious Mind.</u>

My point to you is this: Don't forsake the inner world of thoughts and belief systems. While fasting, take a deep, searching inventory of the thoughts and beliefs that you have about yourself. Remember: The battle is in the mind. That's what makes techniques as *The Time Trap Escape* and *Detox Breathing* are so effective. So take your time and search your mind and heart for any hidden poisonous thoughts and belief systems that may be trying to sabotage all of your hard work. Ok, here's the action path laid out for you:

* Start the 14-day pre-fast diet to kickstart weight loss and detoxification, paying close attention to all of the banned foods listed. Use the sample menus to cook clean and light meals for yourself during those 14 days. If your digestive system is highly toxic, you can try one or two tablets of Herbs & Prunes.

* Start a fasting journal and write in it what goes through your mind and heart, before, during and after the fast. The journal should go with you wherever you go. When hunger and detox symptoms strike, take it out and write what you are feeling (*use profanity if necessary*). Dump it all in your journal!

* Download the Fasting Masterclass and save all of the content to a folder on your desktop or my documents called *'fasting-masterclass'*.
(http://www.fitnessthroughfasting.com/pos

t-purchase-thanks.html)

*Learn how the <u>Time Trap Escape</u>, <u>Detox Breathing</u>, seltzer water, green tea, chamomile tea, tryptophan and valerian root can help you to confront and overcome hunger and detox symptoms so that you can go the distance. **TTE** and Detox Breathing are very effective, but you must take the time to practice them. If at first you don't get it, continue and do **NOT** give up on these tools!

*Candidly begin to answer the <u>'anchor questions'</u> designed to strengthen your willpower and determination. Consistently expand your answers, write at greater depth **WHY** doing this is important to you and how you will feel if you make it, as well as how you will feel if you don't do it. The more detail and emotion you put into answering those anchor questions, the more effective they will be to help you fight off hunger, detox symptoms and discouragement.

*Complete the 14-day Pre-Fast Diet and choose a start date for the 30-day water fast. This is Phase One of the process; it sets the foundation by cutting out junk, reducing portions and initiating the weight loss and detoxification process. Done properly, the pre-fast diet will reduce the intensity of hunger and detox symptoms once you start water fasting.

*Launch the 30-day water fast, utilizing all of the internal and external tools that you've learned to overcome hunger and detox symptoms.

Consistently listen to the masterclass material, and visit the Fasting Forum and do at least two posts daily to interact with other people who are fasting. Furthermore, speak to your **DESIGNATE** person at the very least three times weekly.

*Read the daily motivational messages, spend time doing your customary devotionals, write, write and write some more in your journal! Constantly recite the *'warrior's mindset'* to fill your mind with optimism, motivation and inspiration.

*Complete 30 days of water fasting. Immediately read and carry out the *'breaking a fast'* instructions, paying attention to follow it for *10 days* exactly as outlined.

*After day 10 of breaking a fast, jump

directly into **The Permanent Weight Loss Diet** as your long-term, structured diet. Take care to study the enclosed charts, shopping lists and menus so that you can get a clear picture of how this diet works.

*Make a commitment with yourself that you will stick to this diet for at least six-to-nine months, so as to give your body sufficient time to lose more fat, stabilize its weight and completely heal, cleanse and rejuvenate.

This is a lot of work, but it is crucial and it is doable. You have everything that you need in this book to lose weight, detoxify and transform your health. All that remains is for you to jump into the water and start swimming. Are you ready? If, on the other hand, you have tried but were not able to complete the entire fast, please don't worry. Yes, I know – it is a tough call. But it is not impossible. Just because you were unable to complete it on one particular try, that doesn't mean that you failed.

This distinction is crucial because it is at this point that many people give up. They feel that losing weight is too hard or impossible. That is simply **NOT TRUE**!

You are continuing to learn and position yourself for breakthrough. This process is challenging but highly rewarding. So do not be discouraged. Progress, not perfection – is the key! **If You Fall Off The Wagon, Stop!** Identify the foods that caused you to stumble. What happened? What caused you to reach for the wrong food? Write about it in the journal. You can be certain that whichever food you ate is likely in the *'banned'* list, right? It isn't the end of the world. This process is, in many ways, like working out. If you are out of shape, at first you probably won't be able to lift much weight.

But, if you are persistent and keep at it, little by little you will get better at it. Losing weight and learning to eat is like mastering any task. If you have been overweight for a long time, you have to also confront the emotional addiction that we have to many of these foods.

The more you practice *water fasting, breaking the fast* and then adopting *The Permanent Weight Loss Diet*, the more all of this will fade and the closer you will get to your ultimate goal. I can guarantee you that this is the truth because such was the case with me. So don't ever give up. Keep moving forward!

God bless and Godspeed!

ROBERT DAVE JOHNSTON

To access the Fasting Masterclass, go to:

http://www.fitnessthroughfasting.com/post-purchase-thanks.html

To access the Fasting Forum, go to:

http://forum.fitnessthroughfasting.com

Grab The Entire Collection!

How to Lose Weight Fast, Keep it Off & Renew the Mind, Body & Spirit Through Fasting, Smart Eating & Practical Spirituality

Volume 1: The 'Permanent Weight Loss' Diet

Volume 2: The Intermittent Fasting Weight Loss Formula

Volume 3: How to Lose 30 Pounds (Or More) In 30 Days with Juice Fasting

Volume 4: Burn the Blubber; How to Lose Belly Fat Fast, and For Good!

Volume 5: Lose the Emotional Baggage: Transform Your Mind & Spirit with Fasting

Volume 6: How to Break a Fast and Keep the Weight Off

Volume 7: How to Lose 40 Pounds (Or More) in 30 Days with Water Fasting

Volume 8: Compilation Volumes 1-6 -> Get All 6 For The Price Of 4!

Also by Robert Dave Johnston:

Binge Free – Triumph Over Binge Eating, Confessions of a Former Food Addict, Volume 1

How to Lose Weight & Keep it Off by Transforming the Mind & Behaviors

Volume 1: How to Lose Weight & Keep it Off By Reprogramming the Subconscious Mind

Volume 2: Mental Strategies to Defeat Diet Hunger and Junk Food Cravings

Volume 3: The Cravings Ninja Assassin

Volume 4: How to Cheat On Your Diet (And Get Away With It)

Volume 5: Compilation

Detoxify Your Body, Lose Weight, Get Healthy & Transform Your Life

Volume 1: The 10-Day 'At-Home' Colon Cleansing Formula

Volume 2: Bug Off! A 30-Day Parasite, Liver, Kidney Detox & Weight Loss Plan

Volume 3: Lose 30 Pounds (Or More) in 30 Days with Intermittent Fasting & Coffee Enemas

Volume 4: Compilation: Get All 3 for the Price of 2

Don't forget to check the articles and growing health community at: FitnessThroughFasting.com

Rob's first work of horror/fiction has just been released.

The King of Pain – A Journey to Hell & Back Through the Mind's Eye Volume 1 – The Descent

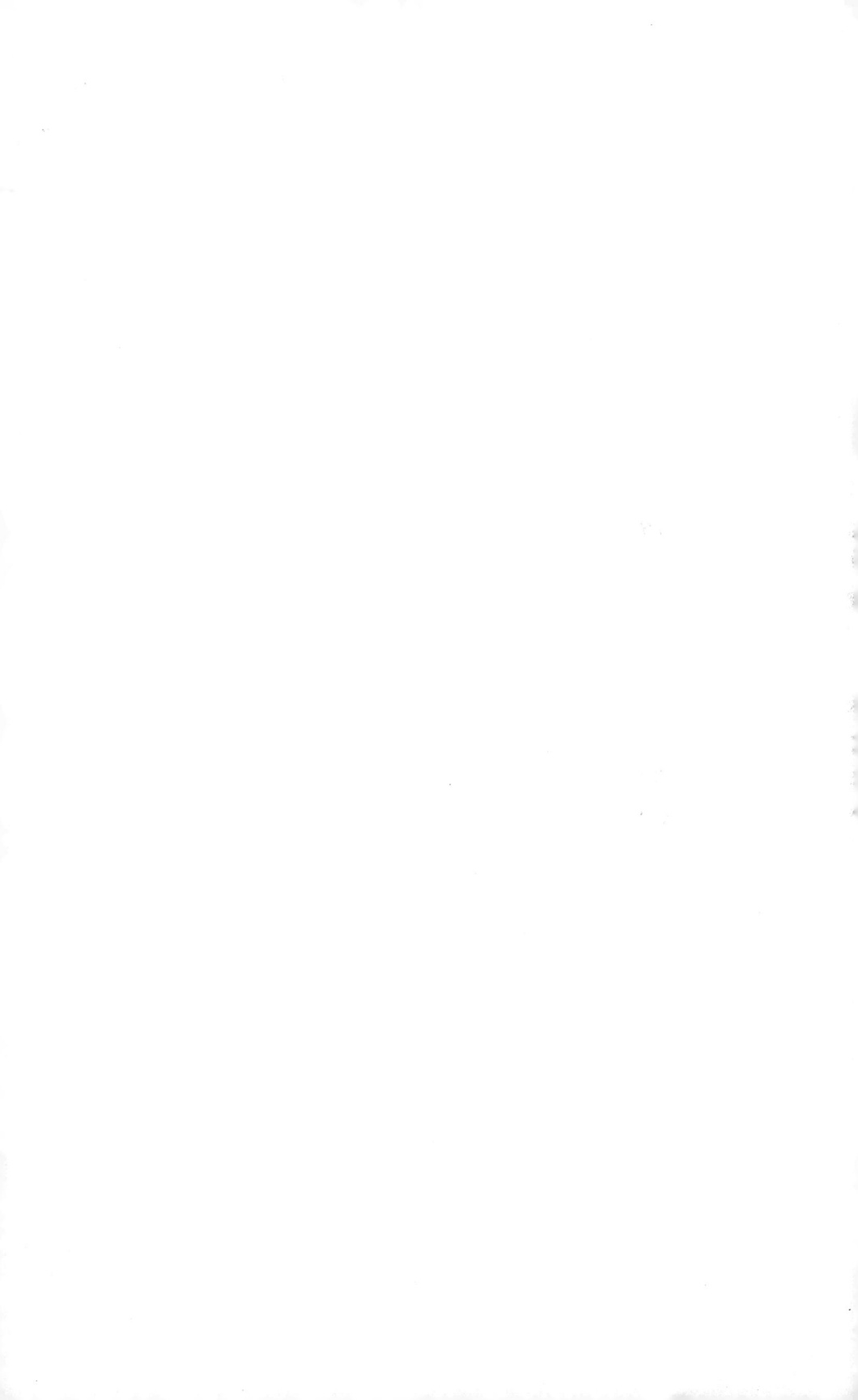

Printed in Great Britain
by Amazon